FEVER

FEVER

ITS BIOLOGY, EVOLUTION, AND FUNCTION

Matthew J. Kluger

PRINCETON UNIVERSITY PRESS
PRINCETON, NEW JERSEY

Published by Princeton University Press, Princeton, New Jersey.
In the United Kingdom: Princeton University Press, Guildford, Surrey.

Library of Congress Cataloging in Publication Data will be found on the last printed page of this book.

This book has been composed in VIP Baskerville.

Clothbound editions of Princeton University Press books are printed on acid-free paper, and binding materials are chosen for strength and durability.

Printed in the United States of America by Princeton University Press, Princeton, New Jersey.

For Susan,
Sharon, and Hilary

Contents

List of Tables

List of Figures

Acknowledgments

Many people have read and commented on various aspects of this book. For their time-consuming, careful, and important efforts, I thank my wife Susan Kluger, and my friends and colleagues Eric Rabkin, Richard Gonzalez, and Laurie Hoffman-Goetz. Thanks also go to Barbara Rothenburg for her careful proofreading of the manuscript and to Wendell Goetz for his translation of Liebermeister's works. I also thank Betty Martin for typing the finished manuscript.

There is one other person who contributed significantly to the production of this book—Horace W. Davenport. In my six years in the Department of Physiology at the University of Michigan, I have been free to pursue my own research and scholarly interests regardless of whether they have been along the "main line" of medical school physiology. It was only in this type of atmosphere that much of the work described in this book could have been performed. For H.W.D.'s philosophy of allowing each faculty member to pursue his own special area of interest in an environment conducive to intellectual development, I am especially grateful.

Thanks go to the following authors and publishers for allowing me to reproduce their figures:

Figure 2. Courtesy of Cambridge University Press.

Figure 4. Courtesy of D. Gates, Harper and Row Press.

Figure 6. Courtesy of K. Nagy, *Science*. Copyright 1972 by the American Association for the Advancement of Science.

Figures 7 and 8. Courtesy of Columbia University Press.

Figure 9. Courtesy of G. Fraenkel, Dover Publications.

Figure 10. Courtesy of B. Heinrich, *American Scientist*.

Figure 14. Courtesy of B. Hellstrom, *American Journal of Physiology*.

Figure 16. Courtesy of J. Hayward, American Elsevier Publications.

Figure 17. Courtesy of *The American Journal of Physiology*.

Figure 20. Courtesy of J. Bligh, Elsevier/North Holland Biomedical Press.

Figure 21. Courtesy of M. Cabanac, *Journal of Physiology* (London).

Figure 25. Courtesy of P. Beeson, *Journal of Experimental Medicine*.

Figures 26 and 27. Courtesy of J. Splawinski, Pflugers Archiv.

Figure 28. Courtesy of E. Atkins, *Yale Journal of Biology and Medicine*.

Figure 29. Courtesy of R. Good, *The Journal Lancet* (Minneapolis).

Figure 30. Courtesy of W. Cranston, *Journal of Physiology* (London).

Figure 31. Courtesy of H. Laburn, *Journal of Physiology* (London).

Figure 32. Courtesy of H. Hensel, Pflugers Archiv.

Figure 33. Courtesy of The University of Chicago Press.

Figures 34 and 35. Courtesy of the *Journal of Physiology* (London).

Figures 37 and 38. Courtesy of the *American Journal of Physiology*.

Figure 39. Courtesy of the *Journal of Physiology* (London).

Figures 42 and 43. Courtesy of L. Vaughn, *Journal of Physiology* (London).

Figure 45. Courtesy of *Science*. Copyright 1975 by the American Association for the Advancement of Science

Figure 46. Courtesy of *Science*. Copyright 1976 by the American Association for the Advancement of Science.

Figure 47. Courtesy of W. Reynolds, *Nature*.

Figure 48. Courtesy of G. Nahas, Society for Experimental Biology and Medicine.

Introduction

Fever has long been recognized as a symptom of disease. Until about 100 years ago, it seems that fever was considered to be a healthy sign during disease; but by the late 1800s this view began to change, and the use of antipyretic drugs to reduce fevers became commonplace.

It has been difficult to obtain data pertinent to the question of whether fever has a beneficial or harmful effect on an infected host. As the result of indirect evidence, it has often been assumed that fever has survival value. This is because fever is an energetically costly process. As a febrile organism elevates its body temperature, it consumes considerably more energy, simply as the result of the effects of temperature on biochemical or metabolic processes. This has led to the conclusion that this process would not have evolved had it no adaptive function.

What about hard experimental data? Conceptually, one way to resolve whether fever is adaptive would be to infect a group of mammals with some harmful bacteria or virus and then allow one half to develop a normal fever and prevent the other half from raising their body temperatures. The survival of the two populations of mammals would be compared and if fever were harmful, then the group which was prevented from elevating its body temperature would have a greater survival rate. If fever were beneficial, then the opposite results would be obtained. The problem with this experiment is that it is very difficult to attentuate the fever in an infected group of mammals without making the results difficult to interpret. In the process of preventing the fever, one must administer antipyretic drugs or perform some other manipulation which would confound the results. For example, would the differences in the survival rate of the two populations be attributable to the effects of the drugs on body temperature or to some side effect not related to their antipyretic properties? There have, nevertheless, been many experiments, using mammals, which have attempted to resolve whether fever is adaptive or maladaptive, and while the results of these studies are difficult to interpret, they tend to indicate that in many cases fever is beneficial to the infected host.

Another approach to determining the function of fever has been to find a more appropriate animal to use in one's investigations. This really becomes a question of selecting the best animal to use to answer a specific question. For example, if one is interested in the effects of some drug on the cardiovascular system, then one often uses the dog or the laboratory rabbit as the experimental animal. One advantage is that they are large and, therefore, relatively easy to work with. Another and perhaps more important advantage is that since their cardiovascular system is similar to that of human beings, the results obtained using these animals can often be extrapolated to other vertebrates, including man. Neurobiology is another area in which the proper selection of an experimental animal has produced important results. When one is interested in some aspect of nerve cell function, cells from invertebrates, such as the squid, are often used. These cells are often selected because they are large and easily accessible. Furthermore, since the physiology of nerve cells tends to be relatively conservative from one group of animals to another, the results obtained using the nerve cells of most invertebrates can be extrapolated to basic nerve processes in other groups of organisms. The scientific literature is literally filled with the fruitful results obtained by investigators who carefully selected the most appropriate animal species for their investigations.

It seemed to us that one way to resolve the question of the role of fever in disease would be to use an ectothermic organism as the experimental animal. An ectotherm (in contrast to an endotherm) is an organism which regulates its body temperature largely by behavioral processes. Reptiles, amphibians, and fishes are examples of ectothermic vertebrates. If these organisms developed fevers in response to infection, then one would have an excellent experimental animal to use to investigate fever's function. Such an animal could be infected with live pathogenic organisms, and because its body temperature could be easily controlled by the experimenter, it would be possible to investigate the effects of holding the animal at febrile and afebrile body temperatures.

First, we had to determine whether ectotherms developed fevers in response to infection. If they did, this by itself would provide indirect evidence that fever was beneficial, for why else would fever be found in vertebrates from fishes through mammals? As a result, a series of experiments was initiated to trace the evolution of fever. Much of this book is a summary of these investigations, by members of my laboratory and others, to trace the evolution and to investigate the adaptive value of fever.

This book is divided into four chapters. The first chapter introduces the subject of regulation of body temperature. In this chapter, temperature regulation is discussed as a reflex containing sensors, integrators, and effectors. The major point of this chapter is that in both endotherms and ectotherms, the sensors and integrators are similar, and therefore the primary difference between endotherms and ectotherms resides in the effector side of this reflex.

In the second chapter the biology of fever is discussed. During a fever, the organism behaves as though its thermoregulatory set-point has been elevated and as a result, it actively raises its body temperature by using both physiological and behavioral means. This chapter argues that since pyrogens (fever inducing agents) affect either the sensors or integrators of temperature regulation, both endotherms and ectotherms should develop fevers in response to infection. The third chapter largely reviews the results obtained in my laboratory as well as those in the laboratories of Dr. W. Reynolds and J. Covert of the Pennsylvania State University concerning the evolution of the febrile response. The final chapter discusses our present understanding of the role of fever in disease. This last chapter includes both a critical review of the literature prior to 1960 and a summary of the more recent findings concerning fever's function.

FEVER

1. Regulation of Body Temperature in the Vertebrates

Why Regulate Body Temperature?

The energy expended by "warm-blooded" organisms, such as ourselves, to regulate our body temperature is enormous: temperature regulation is costly. For example, at low environmental temperatures, people might have to expend 1800 kcal/day, or more, solely to generate the heat necessary to maintain a body temperature of 37°C and perhaps 10% more at febrile temperatures. This expenditure of energy often amounts to over 90% of the total energy used in any given day for performing external work. The energy, of course, comes from the food we eat, and as a result, we must eat an equivalent amount of kcal of food each day just to regulate body temperature. On days when our food intake falls below our daily energy expenditure, we rely on our stores of fat for this source of energy, resulting in a loss of weight. One can calculate, approximately, the amount of energy saved by a resting human-sized organism which does not regulate its body temperature, and therefore remains at a constant environmental temperature, say 20°C. This organism would have a metabolic rate (energy expenditure) roughly equivalent to that of the American alligator, or about 60 kcal/day (Altman and Dittmer 1974). In other words, regulating can cost about thirty times more than not regulating body temperature (1800 kcal/day vs. 60 kcal/day).

Expending and therefore procuring such large amounts of energy have led to numerous adaptations in birds, mammals, and other "warm-blooded" organisms. These adaptations have increased the efficiency of these organisms to obtain, digest, and utilize large volumes of food. Based on the enormous energy cost of regulating body temperature, it is often speculated that there must be some adaptive value in maintaining body temperature at a high and fairly constant level rather than allowing body temperature to fluctuate with the environmental temperature. The adaptive value of regulating body temperature is thought to be related to the effect of temperature on biochemical reactions.

The physiology of any organism can ultimately be reduced to a series of chemical reactions. Most of these reactions are strongly influenced by temperature. The effect of increasing temperature on the rate of increase in biochemical reactions is often greater than can be explained simply by the thermally induced increase in the average kinetic energy of the reacting molecules. For example, many biochemical reactions increase their reaction rate two to threefold over a 10°C rise in temperature (this is often referred to as a "Q_{10}" of 2 or 3). Based on simple molecular kinetics, a 10°C rise in temperature should have increased the reaction rate only a few percent (Giese 1968). In the late 1800s, the Swedish physical chemist Arrhenius proposed that the often logarithmic increase in the reaction rates of biochemical reactions is related to their activation energy. Arrhenius mathematically characterized the effects of temperature on biochemical reactions, pointing out that most biochemical reactions tend to increase logarithmically with increasing temperature to a point of maximization. Above this optimal temperature, the reactions decrease (Johnson et al. 1954). Examples of this profound effect temperature has on biological systems can be seen in its effect on the growth rates of various organisms (Figures 1-3).

Organisms which regulate their body temperature maintain a degree of biochemical stability not found in the nonthermoregulators. Not only have their biochemical reactions evolved to function optimally at or near the regulated body temperature, but, perhaps more importantly, these reactions can now occur in comparative independence of the environmental temperature. A normal reduction in the environmental temperature does not slow the metabolic processes of a thermoregulator like a bird or mammal.

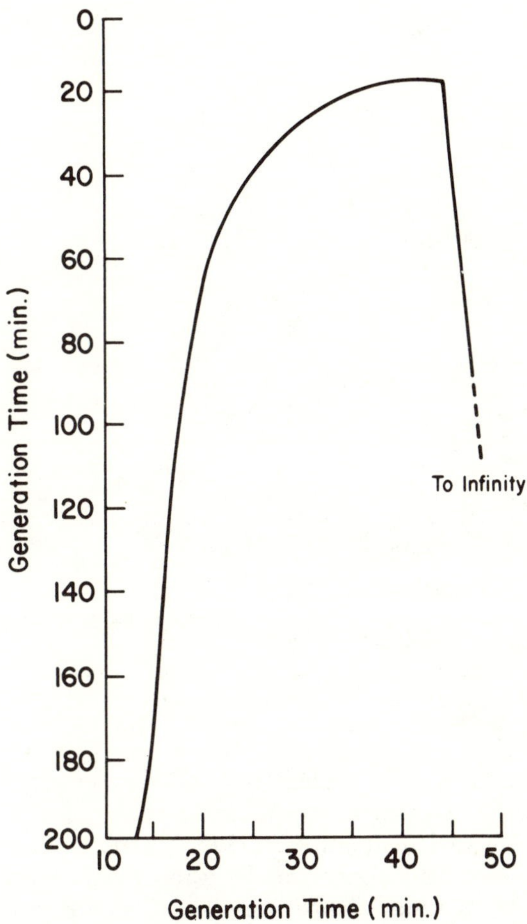

Figure 1. Effect of environmental temperature on the generation time of *E. coli* bacteria. Note that the shortest time between generations is around 40°C, the so-called optimum temperature for growth for this species of bacterium. (Data redrawn from Barber 1908.)

Birds, mammals, and representatives from some other groups of organisms are thermoregulators called "endotherms." Endotherms have the capability of internally generating sufficient amounts of heat to raise their body temp-

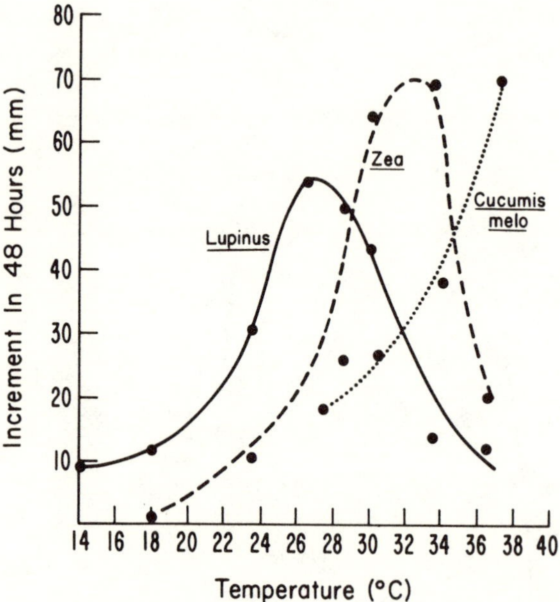

Figure 2. Effect of temperature on the rate of growth of common plants indigenous to temperate (*Lupinus*) and warmer climates (*Zea* and *Cucumis melo*). (Based on D'Arcy Thompson 1942; data of Sachs.)

erature considerably above the environmental temperature. Endotherms have been freed, to some extent, from the effects of environmental temperature. They can remain active, maintaining optimal conditions for their biochemical reactions, over a wide range of environmental temperatures. Subtle changes in environmental temperature which would markedly affect the biochemical reactions of nonthermoregulators do not affect endotherms.

There is another group of thermoregulators which, unlike the endotherms, lack the metabolic machinery to generate internally large quantities of heat—the ectotherms. Reptiles, fishes, and representatives from many other groups of animals are ectotherms. An ectotherm relies primarily on behavioral adjustments to maintain a fairly constant body

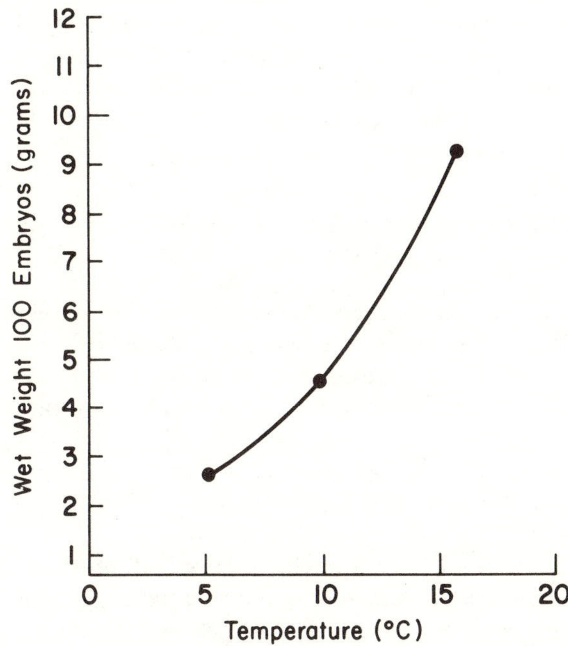

Figure 3. Effect of temperature on the rate of growth of trout larvae. Weights were taken at sixty days after fertilization. (Data based on Gray 1928.)

temperature. A lizard such as the desert iguana, for example, regulates its body temperature at 39°C ± 1°C by moving into the sunlight when its body temperature falls below 38°C and into the shade when its body temperature rises above 40°C. This form of thermoregulation, which is energetically cheaper than generating the heat internally, nonetheless provides the advantages of biochemical stability found in the endotherms. However, the ectotherm can only regulate its body temperature in environments which have the appropriate thermal profile. At night, on overcast days, or during the winter, the ectotherm "slows down" as its body temperature falls toward the environmental temperature.

The regulation of body temperature, therefore, allows an organism to maintain a thermodynamically stable internal environment in which increases or decreases in the rates of millions of individual biochemical reactions can be changed by the organism (by changing the concentrations of enzymes or substrates) without the need to compensate for changes in environmental temperature.

Why is Body Temperature of Thermoregulators Generally between 35° and 42°C?

It is a curious fact that most terrestrial temperature regulators do their regulating somewhere between 35° and 42°C. Theoretically, a terrestrial thermoregulator could have evolved a system to maintain a reasonably constant body temperature at 5°C or perhaps even 95°C, temperatures substantially above and below the freezing and boiling points of body fluids, respectively. But why within 35° to 42°C?

The upper thermal limit for the survival of most organisms is about 45°C. Above this temperature, proteins tend to denature (lose their tertiary structure). Thus, the thermoregulators are often within a few degrees of their upper lethal limit. The explanation for the regulation of body temperature generally within 10°C of this upper lethal limit is thought to be related to the effects of temperature on biochemical reactions, to the physics of heat exchange between an organism and the environment, and to the average temperature of the earth.

To regulate body temperature at any given level, an organism's rate of heat gain (sum of rate of heat absorbed from the environment + rate of internal heat production) must equal its rate of heat loss. When these are out of balance, body temperature will rise or fall

$$\text{Heat Gain} = \text{Heat Loss} \tag{1}$$

depending on which side of equation (1) is greater. Heat is exchanged between an organism and its environment by four physical processes: conduction, convection, radiation, and evaporation. These forms of energy exchange will be described briefly.

1. Conduction. When I touch the metal bookcase in my office, it feels colder than the surrounding air temperature. This is because air is a poor conductor of heat (a good insulator) and metal is a good conductor of heat (a poor insulator). Heat flows from my hand, which might be at 32°C, to the metal bookcase, which might be at 22°C, by a process known as conduction. Heat, which flows from a higher to a lower temperature, is passed directly to the bookcase. The temperature of my hand will fall as the result of this transfer of heat; the temperature of the bookcase will rise. The process of heat transfer by conduction occurs by the movement of heat energy between adjacent molecules and occurs without any mass motion in the medium through which this energy is moving. Conduction of heat can be represented by the following equation:

$$K/t = A\frac{k}{L}(T_1 - T_2) \qquad (2)$$

where, K = conductive heat exchange
t = time
A = area
L = distance between T_1 and T_2
k = coefficient of conductivity
T_1 and T_2 = temperatures of two objects

This equation asserts that the rate of conductive heat transfer between two objects is related to the surface area in contact, the distance the heat must travel, the thermal conductivities of the substances, and the difference in temperature between the two objects. If the metal bookcase were at a temperature above my hand's temperature, then clearly heat would be gained from the bookcase and my hand's temperature would rise.

2. Convection. Heat is also lost from our bodies by the transfer of heat from our skin surface to the fluid medium which surrounds us, this medium being either air or water. The rate of heat lost by convection can be represented by the following equation:

$$C/t = c\,A\,(T_1 - T_2) \qquad (3)$$

where, C = convective heat exchange
t = time
c = convective heat transfer coefficient
A = area
T_1 and T_2 = temperatures of two objects

As in conductive heat loss, convective heat exchange is proportional to the area in contact with, in this case, the medium, and to the difference in temperature between the two objects. It is also dependent upon the coefficient of convection. The coefficient of convection is related to the type of medium in which the exchange of heat is occurring, and the velocity of movement of the medium, as well as other charcteristics. The increase in convective heat loss on windy days (c increases) is a well-known phenomenon and goes into forming the commonly used wind-chill index to describe the subjective sensation of coldness.

3. Radiation. All objects above absolute zero (−273°C) emit energy in the form of radiation. We are constantly gaining and losing heat by radiation based on the following equation:

$$R/t = \sigma e_1 e_2 A\,(T_1^4 - T_2^4) \qquad (4)$$

where, R = radiant heat exchange
t = time
σ = Stefan-Boltzmann constant
e_1, e_2 = emissivities of the radiating objects
A = area
T_1, T_2 = temperatures of radiating objects (in absolute temperature)

Without even attempting to describe in any detail the significance of σ, or the emissivities of the radiating objects, one can see that the rate of heat exchange by radiation is, as in conduction and convection, related to the area and to the difference in temperature between the two objects (in this case to the fourth power of the absolute temperature).

For our purposes, the key point about conduction, convection, and radiation is that they are all dependent upon a difference in temperature. Heat flows from a higher temperature to a lower temperature.

4. Evaporation. Heat is lost from our bodies by evaporation of water from our respiratory tract or from our skin (sweating). During periods of heat stress induced by exercise (an internal heat stress) or by exposure to high environmental temperatures, we can lose a liter or more of sweat each hour. Each liter of sweat which evaporates from our skin surface removes approximately 580 kcal (latent heat of vaporization of water at skin temperature). Sweating is, therefore, an enormously effective mechanism for losing heat. The rate of heat lost by evaporation is given by equation (5):

$$E/t = A\,b\,(V.P._1 - V.P._2) \tag{5}$$

where, E = heat lost by evaporation
t = time
A = area
b = coefficient of evaporation
$V.P._1$, $V.P._2$ = vapor pressures of surface where water is evaporating and the vapor pressure of the air surrounding that surface

The amount of heat lost by evaporation is related to the area exposed to evaporation, a coefficient of evaporation (which is a function of wind velocity, latent heat of vaporization, and other variables), and the vapor pressure differences between the evaporating surface and the air. When the vapor pressure (or partial pressure) of water on our skin surface is equal to the vapor pressure of the air, then no evaporation occurs. The sweat simply drips off our bodies and does not contribute to cooling us. This is what happens when the relative humidity is 100%. (The relative humidity is defined as the ratio of the environmental vapor pressure to the maximum or saturated vapor pressure at the same temperature.) Under these conditions, the vapor pressure on our skin surface (which is generally close to, or at, the saturated level) equals the saturated vapor pressure of the surrounding air.

Figure 4 summarizes the basics of heat exchange between an organism and its environment. For more detailed accounts of heat exchange, the reader is referred to Carlson and Hsieh (1970), Brengelmann (1973), Gates (1972), Lowry (1967), and Birkebak (1966).

What does this brief introduction to energy exchange between an organism and its environment have to do with the regulation of body temperature between 35° and 42°C? The mean or average temperature of the earth on its surface is about 16°C (Gates 1972). Obviously, temperatures in different areas of the world and at different times of the day and year vary significantly from 16°C; but generally, a thermoregulator will be above the environmental temperature. Let us assume for a moment that an animal regulates its body temperature at 25°C. When the environmental temperature is at the mean earth temperature of 16°C, the heat which the animal produces by its metabolic processes would

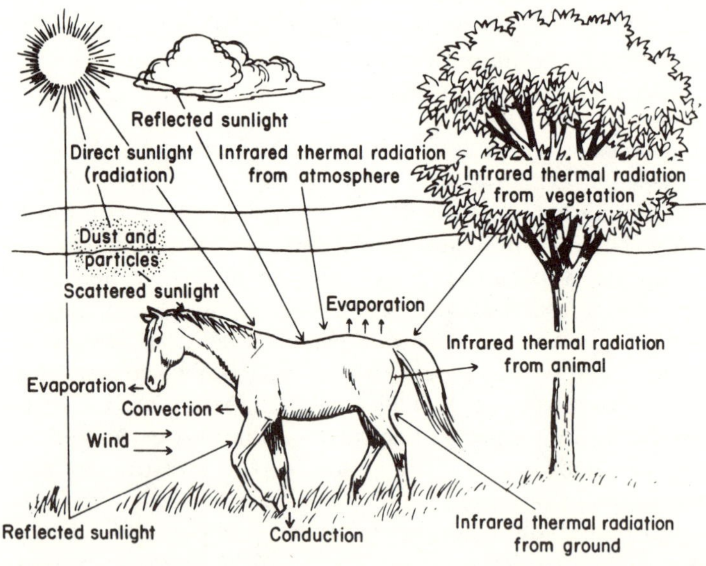

Figure 4. Avenues of heat transfer between an animal and its environment. (Based on Gates 1972.)

be dissipated to the environment by the processes of conduction, convection, radiation, and evaporation. When the environmental temperature is 30°C, a temperature which often occurs during the summer months even in temperate climates, the processes of conduction, convection, and radiation would serve to increase the animal's body temperature. This is because heat would now flow from the higher environmental temperature to the lower temperature of the thermoregulator—see equations (2-4). The animal must now rely entirely on evaporation of water to maintain its temperature at 25°C. Because evaporation of water removes such large quantities of heat, the animal would still face little difficulty regulating its body temperature at 25°C. There are, however, two potential problems involved in relying completely on evaporation as a means of maintaining a constant body temperature. The first occurs for the thermoregulator when water is scarce. In certain areas of the world, perhaps a desert during a summer day, the air temperature might approach 50°C. The hot desert winds tend to warm the individual by convective heat transfer from the environment to the individual. However, since the air is dry, a person regulates his body temperature by the evaporation of water. To maintain a body temperature of 37°C, the individual might have to lose up to nineteen liters of water over a twelve-hour period (Gates 1972). To regulate body temperature at 25°C, under these conditions, would be an impossibility. Clearly, the desert during the heat of a summer day is not an environment which thermoregulators prefer, even those that regulate between 35° and 42°C. This is why so many desert animals are nocturnal. The reliance on the evaporation of water to maintain a constant body temperature will not work effectively for desert dwellers, or for any organisms which may face periodic shortages of water.

The second potential problem for a thermoregulator which must rely on water evaporation occurs during periods of high relative humidity. Recall from equation (5) that when the air surrounding the animal becomes as saturated as the surface from which the water must evaporate, evaporation does not occur. Under these conditions the thermoregulator cannot lose heat by evaporation, and body temperature rises. This is exactly what happens to people when they are exposed to high environmental temperatures in a humid environment. Body heat cannot be lost by conduction, convection, or radiation, nor by evaporation. This is why exercising during these environmental conditions often leads to heat related disorders.

Through the process of evolution, terrestrial thermoregulators have evolved a regulated body temperature generally somewhere between 35° and 42°C, close to their upper thermal limit. In most environments there is an adequate temperature gradient from the thermoregulator to the environment to allow for the processes of conduction, convection, and radiation to rid the body of excess heat. This allows the thermoregulator to maintain a fairly constant body temperature and therefore a fairly constant rate of biochemical reactions. This high body temperature also allows the thermoregulator to generally be more "active" than its nonthermoregulating counterpart which is at a body temperature of, for example, 20°C. When the environmental temperature approaches or is even above the thermoregulator's body temperature, then evaporation of water (providing water is freely available and the relative humidity is low) is generally adequate to maintain a relatively stable body temperature. Clearly, a terrestrial thermoregulator maintaining a 20°C or 25°C body temperature would often face environmental conditions where the regulation of body temperature would be impossible.

Origins of Temperature Regulation

Although this chapter is primarily aimed at introducing the reader to temperature regulation in the vertebrates, I think it is interesting to explore briefly the question of the evolution of temperature regulation. Somewhat surprisingly, there are representatives from diverse life forms that regulate their body temperature. To place the regulation of body temperature in the vertebrates into proper perspective, I have selected three examples from remotely related groups which also regulate their body temperature.

A. Plant Thermoregulation

We generally think of the temperature of plants as being roughly equal to that of their environment. As the environmental temperature rises, so does the temperature of the plant, resulting in an increase in the plant's metabolic activities. There is, however, a large group of monocotyledonous plants, members of the arum family (Aracae) which have representatives that regulate their temperature (Meeuse 1966; Nagy et al. 1972; Knutson 1974). The arum family contains such familiar plants as the philodendron (*Philodendron selloum*), skunk cabbage (*Symplocarpus foetitus*), and jack-in-the-pulpit (*Arisaema sp.*) (Figure 5). One of the characteristics of this family is the possession of a long reproductive organ called a spadix. The spadix emits volatile chemicals which attract insects that pollinate the plants. (One seldom

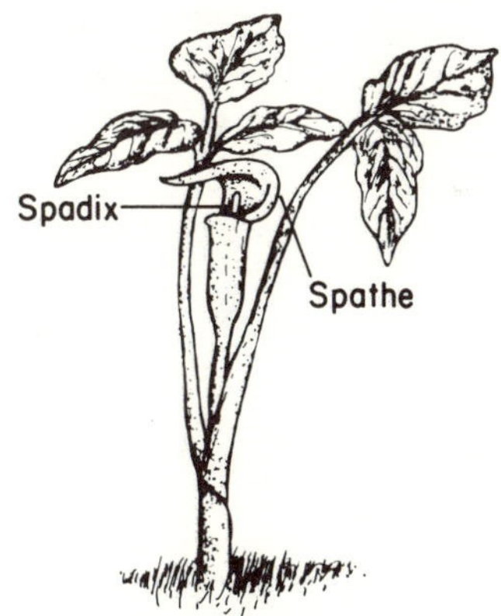

Figure 5. Drawing of the well-known member of the arum family, jack-in-the-pulpit. Note the long spadix surrounded by the leaflike structure known as the spathe. In some members of this family, such as in skunk cabbages and philodendrons, the spadix regulates its temperature when in bloom. To the author's knowledge, it is not presently known whether the spadix of jack-in-the-pulpit regulates its temperature when blooming.

sees a spadix on the common household varieties of philodendron as they seldom reach reproductive maturity in the artificial environment found in most homes.) During periods of flowering, for several hours each day (in the philodendron) or for periods of greater than two weeks (in skunk cabbage), the spadix remains as much as 30°C or more above the environmental temperature (Figure 6). Concurrent with this elevated and regulated spadix temperature is a rise in the metabolic activity of the spadix. As the environmental temperature falls, the oxygen consumption of the spadix rises, resulting in an increase in its heat production. The responses of the spadix to changes in environmental temperature are similar to those found in small mammals and birds.

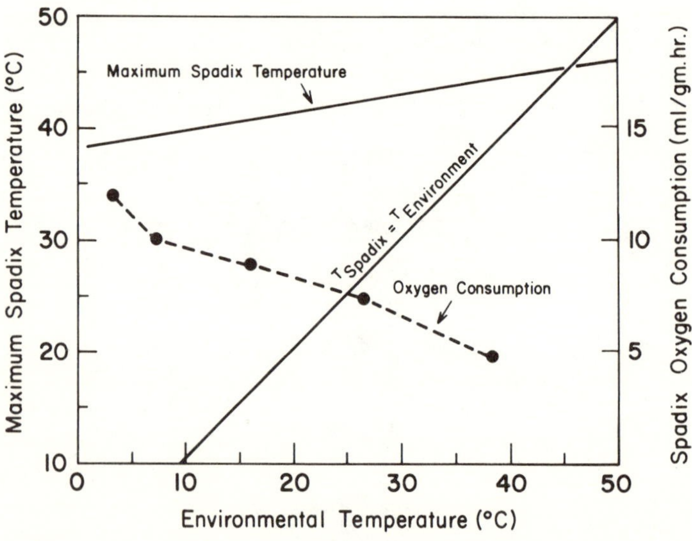

Figure 6. Maximum core temperature and oxygen consumption of the spadices of the common garden philodendron in various environmental temperatures. Notice that at low environmental temperatures the metabolic activity of the spadix (oxygen consumption) more than doubles. This increased metabolic heat production allows the spadix to maintain a temperature, in some cases, of more than 25°C above the environmental temperature. (Redrawn from Nagy et al. 1972.)

It has been speculated that the regulation of the spadix temperature at a level considerably above environmental temperature during flowering increases the rate of vaporization of insect-attracting chemicals and results in the increased likelihood of cross-fertilization (Meeuse 1966; Nagy et al. 1972).

B. Protozoan Thermoregulation

If Paramecia (common ciliated protozoans) are placed on a glass slide, covered with a glass cover slip, and heated to between 40° and 45°C, one can observe through a microscope active, seemingly random, locomotion. If a drop of cold water is placed on the upper surface of the cover glass, after a short period of time, the Paramecia will be observed congregating under the cold water, thereby avoiding the heated areas of the slide (Jennings 1906). If Paramecia are placed in a trough in which the temperature is maintained constant at about 19°C, they become randomly dispersed (Mendelssohn 1902). If a temperature gradient of 26° to 38°C is established in this trough, the Paramecia are observed congregating close to the 26°C region. If the temperature gradient is from 10° to 25°C then, again, the Paramecia are found near 25°C (Figure 7). Mendelssohn found that the "preferred" temperature of Paramecia is between 24° and 28°C.

The manner by which these ectothermic organisms regulate their body temperature is quite interesting. If one end of the trough is heated beyond the "preferred" temperature, the protozoans in that area become more active, darting about in all directions. Individuals that are swimming toward the hotter end display what has been called the "avoiding reaction" (Figure 8). These series of rotations followed by forward movements are continued until the direction of movement leads the protozoans toward the cooler region. At that point the avoiding reaction ceases and the organisms continue to swim in that general direction. A similar, albeit slower, series of reactions happens at temperatures below the "preferred" temperatures of these protozoans. Thus, after being exposed to either hot or cold tem-

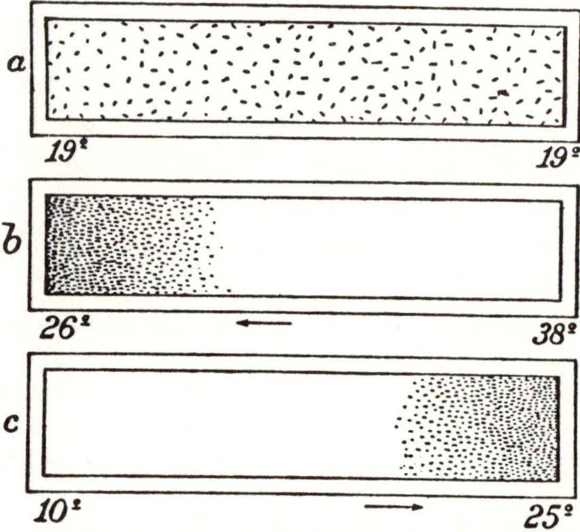

Figure 7. Reactions of Paramecia to heat and cold, after Mendelssohn (1902). At *a* the Paramecia are placed in a trough, both ends of which have a temperature of 19°C. They are scattered equally. At *b* the temperature of one end is raised to 38°C while the other is only 26°C. The Paramecia collect at the end having the lower temperature. At *c*, one end has a temperature of 25°C, while the other is lowered to 10°C. The animals now collect at the end having the higher temperature. (Jennings 1906.)

peratures, the general orientation of most of the protozoans is toward their "preferred" temperature. Protozoan thermoregulation is therefore the result of avoidance of temperature extremes, rather than the active selection of a specific temperature (Jennings 1906). Nevertheless, the net result of these avoidance reactions is the behavioral maintenance of a regulated body temperature.

C. Insect Thermoregulation

The last example of nonvertebrate thermoregulation I will briefly review is that of thermoregulation in insects. The insects have some species which regulate their body temperature by behavioral adjustments (ectotherms) and others that do so by the generation of internal heat (endotherms). Ec-

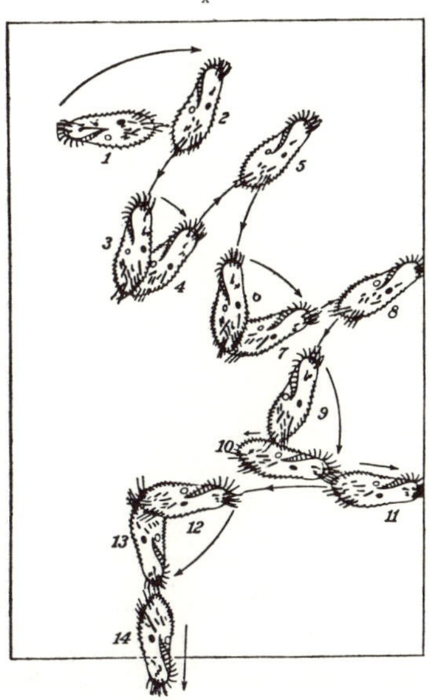

Figure 8. Reaction of the ciliated protozoan *Oxytricha sp.* to heat applied at *x*. The organism moves backward from position 2 to position 3, then swivels on its posterior end to position 4, and then goes forward to position 5. The set of movements 2 to 5 constitutes one turn and is repeated until the organism is in cooler water. When it finally becomes directed away from the heat as at 13-14, it ceases to change its direction of movement and continues to move straight ahead, thus reaching a cooler region. (Jennings 1906.)

tothermy in insects can be illustrated by the response of the desert locust, *Schistocerca gregaria*, to sunlight. In the cool morning air of the desert, the locusts are in a state of cold torpor. As the air temperature warms up to around 17° to 20°C, the locusts slowly begin to move and tend to orient their bodies perpendicular to the sun's rays (Fraenkel and Gunn 1961) (Figure 9). James E. Heath and his associates have shown that this basking behavior serves to substantially increase the rate of warm-up by insects (Heath 1967; Heath and Wilkin 1970; Heath et al. 1971). Once the insects reach a suitably high temperature, they can become more active. Basking behavior leads to an increased level of absorption of radiant energy and actually allows basking insects to main-

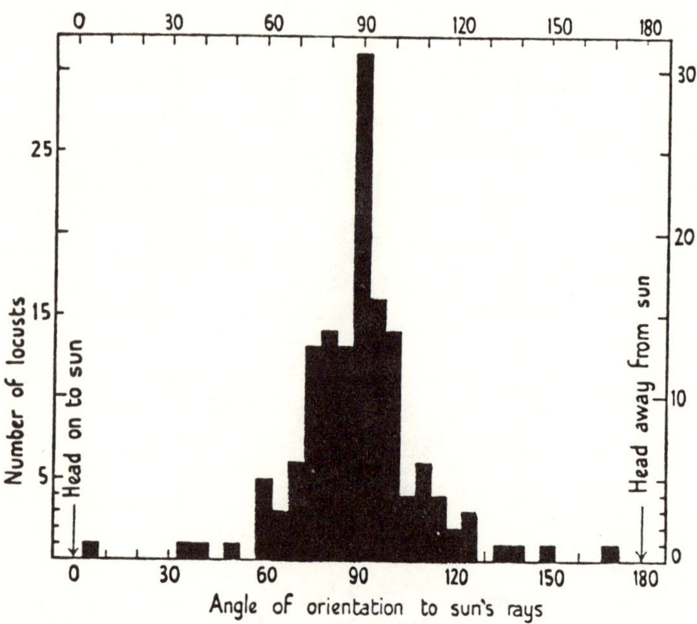

Figure 9. Graph showing the distribution of the angles between the body axes of 142 adult locusts and the projection of the sun's rays on the horizontal. (Based on Fraenkel 1930; from Fraenkel and Gunn 1961.)

tain a body temperature considerably above the environmental temperature. Basking insects not only use behavioral responses to raise body temperature in the morning (or during other cool times of the day or year), but also utilize elaborate behavioral adjustments to prevent overheating. As a result, body temperature during periods of activity is regulated within a fairly narrow range. Some examples of common insects which behaviorally select a temperature range are house flies (*Musca domestica*), blowflies (*Phormia terranovae*), and cicadas (*Magicicada cassini*).

Insects not only rely on behavior to thermoregulate, but some of the larger species (e.g. bees, large moths) can actually generate enough internal heat to regulate their body temperatures by endothermy (Heath and Adams 1965; Heinrich 1974; Heinrich 1977). At rest, a moth or a bumblebee will have a body temperature approximately equal to that of the environmental temperature. Before periods of activity, these insects begin to shiver. Shivering in insects, as in human beings, results in the expenditure of energy without the production of external work (mechanical efficiency equal to 0%). This muscular activity leads to the generation of large quantities of heat. Furthermore, many moths and bees are actually covered with a layer of scales or hair which can reduce heat loss by more than 50% (Church 1960). The extremely high level of metabolic heat production during these warm-up periods, coupled with a reduction in heat loss because of effective insulation, results in a remarkable rate of rise in thoracic temperature. In the bumblebee, for example, thoracic temperature can rise from 24° to 37°C within one minute (Heinrich 1977). At lower environmental temperatures, such as 6°C, this warm-up period may still take as little as fifteen minutes (Figure 10). Once the bee, or moth, has reached this high thoracic temperature, it can then begin to fly. During flight, thoracic temperature is generally regulated to within a few degrees Celsius of its initial flight temperature. The regulation of body temperature in the endothermic insects is strikingly similar to that found in many small mammals and birds (e.g. bats, hummingbirds).

From this brief introduction into the origins of thermoregulation, we can see that thermoregulation is not a charcteristic unique to vertebrates. Not all organisms regulate their body temperature, but, individual species from such remotely related groups as plants, protozoans, and insects have some control over their tissue temperature. Apparently the ability to sense temperature and to respond appropriately in order to regulate tissue temperature must be a phylogenetically ancient characteristic. Clearly a sophisticated nervous system, such as is found in the vertebrates, is not needed to thermoregulate, since plants and single-celled organisms possess this capability. Perhaps this should not be considered all that remarkable knowing the profound effect temperature has on biochemical reactions. With this short introduction to the adaptive value of regulating body temperature, to the manner by which heat is transferred between

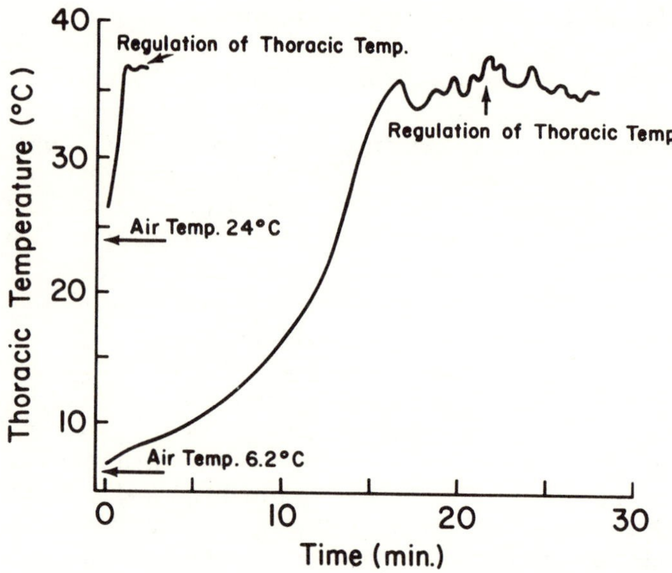

Figure 10. Thoracic temperature changes during and after warm-up in a bumblebee at high and low air temperatures. (Based on Heinrich, 1977.)

the organism and its environment, and to the prevalance of temperature regulation in biological systems, we now turn our attention to the regulation of body temperature in the vertebrates.

Vertebrate Temperature Regulation

The regulation of body temperature can be conceptualized as consisting of the three general components of a reflex arc—1) sensors, 2) integrators, and 3) effectors (Figure 11). The sensors are capable of sensing different temperatures and converting these stimuli into the appropriate signal. In vertebrates, nerve cells serve as temperature sensors. These sensors convert the thermal stimuli into the appropriate patterns and frequencies of action potentials which travel along the afferent or sensory nerves. In vertebrates, temperature sensors have been found in the skin as well as in internal

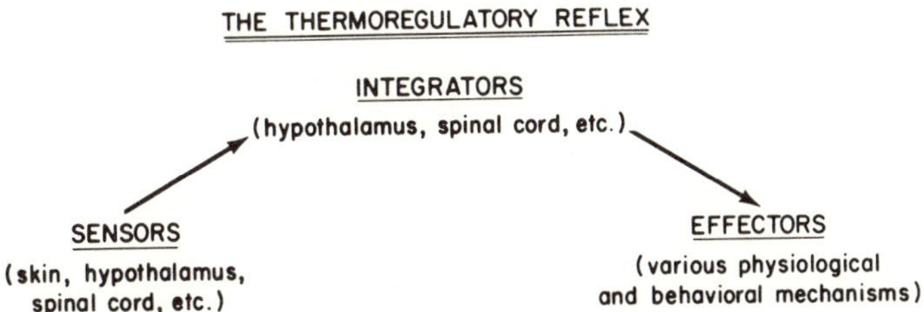

Figure 11. Temperature regulation as a reflex. Sensors located in the skin, spinal cord, hypothalamus, and other areas convey thermal information via nerves to the areas responsible for the integration of temperature. The thermoregulatory integrators, thought to reside primarily in the hypothalamus and spinal cord, send information via efferent nerves and hormones to the thermoregulatory effectors.

structures such as the hypothalamus (a phylogenetically old structure located in the forebrain), spinal cord, and abdomen. The integration of thermal responses in the vertebrates is thought to occur to some extent in the hypothalamus with some integrative abilities residing in other central nervous areas. Here, all the thermal inputs from the various sensors are somehow "weighed" and the appropriate efferent information is then passed on via nerves and hormones to the effectors. The effectors are those structures which actually lead to the raising or lowering of body temperature. Effectors used in regulating body temperature often have other functions as well. Some examples of effectors used by the thermoregulatory system along with their effector response (in parenthesis) are skeletal muscle (shivering; behavioral responses such as moving into or out of the shade), skin blood vessels (increasing or decreasing skin blood flow), sweat glands (sweating), and respiratory system (panting).

Temperature Sensation in the Vertebrates

In vertebrates, the sensation of temperature is accomplished by nerve cells. Little is known about the structure of these nerve receptors. At one time it was thought that specialized encapsulated nerve receptors existed for the sensations of hot and cold (Frey 1895). The temperature receptors which sensed warmth were called "Raffini corpuscles" and those which sensed cold were called "end bulbs of Krause." Even most current histology textbooks still refer to these specialized structures as being responsible for the sensation of temperature in the periphery (skin). A search, however, for a relationship or correlation between these structures and thermal sensitivity proved fruitless (Bligh 1973). It is now thought that specialized hot and cold receptors are simply free nerve endings (Hensel et al. 1973). In the cat, for example, peripheral cold receptors have been identified as the nonmyelinated nerve terminals of myelinated nerve cells (Hensel et al. 1974). (A myelinated nerve cell is one that is surrounded by a sheath of myelin, a protein-lipid layer of electrical insulation; a nonmyelinated nerve cell or segment of nerve cell, in contrast, does not possess this myelin sheath.) The structure of specific warm receptors is as yet unidentified (Hensel et al. 1973). Also unknown is the fundamental mechanism behind a thermoreceptor's ability to transduce or convert thermal energy into a series of action potentials.

Hensel (1974) proposed the following three criteria for a temperature sensor or receptor:

1. The receptor should have a static level of discharge at constant temperatures.
2. The receptor should display a dynamic response to changes in temperature such that warm receptors will increase their frequency of firing (action potentials) with increasing temperature, and cold receptors will increase their rate of firing with decreasing temperature.
3. The receptor should not respond to mild mechanical stimuli by increasing or decreasing its firing frequency.

Thermal receptors which meet the above criteria have been located in the skin, abdomen, veins, hypothalamus, midbrain, and spinal cord (Hensel 1974).

There is a potential problem in relying on the type of information obtained by electrical recordings from nerve cells to categorize temperature sensation in the vertebrates. The problem basically stems from our primitive understanding of the relationship between the patterns or frequencies of action potentials and the actual information used by the living organism. We have no idea whether a neuron that responds to a warm stimulus by increasing its rate or frequency of action potentials actually conveys this information to areas in our brain which are responsible for integrating this thermal information.

More clear-cut results concerning the distribution and quantitative importance of thermal sensors have been obtained in those studies which have actually recorded the animal's physiological and behavioral responses to changes in temperature. These temperature changes can be induced by altering the environmental temperature surrounding the animal (leads to changes in skin temperature), by causing the animal to exercise (leads to an elevation in core temperature), or by selectively heating or cooling a small area of the animal.

We are all aware of the sensations of hot or cold when we exit from an environmentally controlled building. These thermal sensations are presumed to be evidence of peripheral thermal receptors in people. The relative weightings of peripheral temperature sensitive areas in human beings have been investigated by Nadel et al. (1973). They found that the skin on our face possesses about three times the thermal sensitivity as the same area of skin on our chest, abdomen, or thigh. It would be interesting to investigate whether there is a strong correlation between the number(s) of thermally sensitive neurons in these areas and their different thermal sensitivities.

Studies on experimental animals have led to similar findings. For example, when the laboratory rabbit is placed in a cold environment, it maintains a constant body temperature by shivering and other physiological and behavioral mechanisms (Gonzalez et al. 1971). The animal has sensed the cold and reacted accordingly. Peripheral thermal receptors are diffusely located over the skin of the rabbit. Its sparsely furred ears, however, are of particular importance in sensing temperature (Kluger et al. 1971). When the environmental temperature is reduced by 20°C, the skin temperature beneath the thick fur of the back might fall as little as 4° to 5°, whereas the ear skin temperature can fall by as much as 25°C. If these rabbits are placed in the cold, at 8°C, their metabolic heat production increases by about 50%. Warming the ears leads to a decrease in the metabolic heat production and to a concomitant fall in core temperature (Figure 12). These responses occur without any rise in the temperature of the core receptors. Data such as these have shown that the skin is thermally sensitive. In the above example, changing a small area of thermally sensitive tissue actually

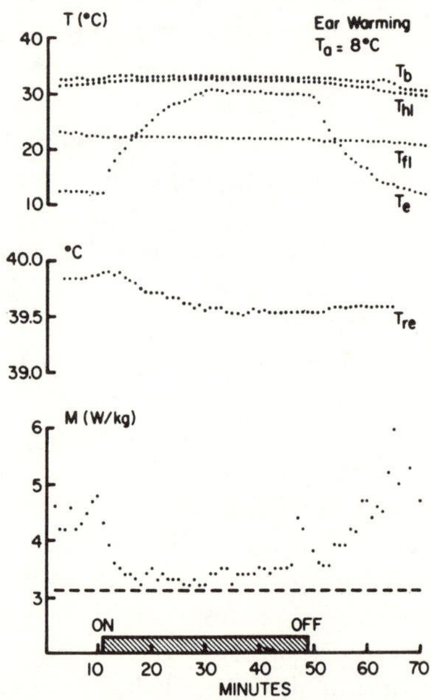

Figure 12. Evidence that heating the ears (T_e) of rabbits in a cool environmental temperature (8°C) leads to a depression in metabolic heat production (M) in watts/kg without a change in other skin temperatures [back (T_b), forelimb (T_{fl}), and hindlimb (T_{hl})]. The dashed line indicates resting metabolism in rabbits at an environmental temperature of 20°C. The decline in M leads to a fall in the rabbit's rectal temperature (T_{re}). (From Kluger et al. 1971.)

leads to changes in core temperature out of proportion with the actual thermal stimulus.

During exercise in a neutral or warm environment, core temperature in birds, mammals, and in some species of fishes and reptiles rises significantly. For example, in flying pigeons, body temperature increases about 2°C (Hart and Roy 1967). Exercising rats and rabbits also increase their body temperature about 2°C (Thompson and Stevenson 1965; Kluger et al. 1973a). Human beings who are exercising often increase their body temperatures by as much as 3°C. These elevations in core temperature are always associated with thermoregulatory effector responses which eventually result in the reestablishment of the preexercise level of body temperature. Core temperature in animals can also be raised artificially. For example, when bats were heated internally with a water-perfused thermode placed in the rectum, body temperature rose several degrees Celsius. When body temperature reached about 37°C, a temperature similar to that encountered during flight, the bats initiated the heat dissipating response of peripheral vasodilation (increasing blood flow to the skin) (Figure 13). As a result of this shunting of warm blood to the skin, skin temperature rose, heat was transferred from the bat to the cooler environment, and core temperature fell (Kluger and Heath 1970). These types of experiments have shown that deep body or core reception of temperature plays an important role in thermoregulation. The locations of these thermoreceptors were, until recently, thought to reside almost totally within the hypothalamus.

Over the past fifty years or so, numerous investigators have manipulated the temperature of discrete areas of the core of animals by using small heating devices called thermodes. A thermode can be simply a wire which is heated by passing current through it. More commonly, however, they are water-perfused stainless steel or polyethylene tubes of varying lengths and diameters (often less than 1 mm). Based on the results of earlier investigators (see the excellent review by Bligh [1973]), it was thought that internal reception of temperature resided primarily in the forebrain, more

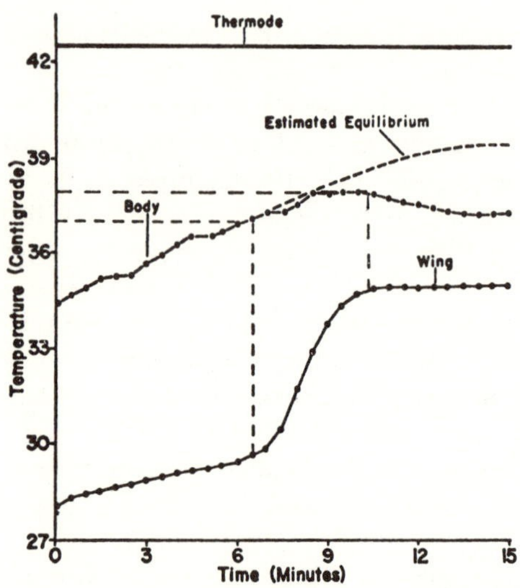

Figure 13. Body and wing temperatures of a bat subjected to constant internal heating (42°-43°C) with a thermode placed into its rectum. Wing temperature is initially about the same as the environmental temperature (28°C). As body temperature rises to above 37°C (6.5 minutes), the wing blood vessels vasodilate and wing temperature rises. Body temperature then declines from 37.9° to 37.2°C. Calculations have shown that if vasodilation had not occurred, the body temperature would have reached 39.5°C. (Based on Kluger and Heath 1970.)

specifically in the anterior hypothalamus and the adjacent preoptic region.

Using a small thermode, the temperature of the hypothalamus of a vertebrate can be raised or lowered without directly affecting other internal temperatures. When the hypothalamic temperature of a dog is raised or lowered as little as 1°C, the dog initiates physiological and behavioral responses which will lead to the lowering or raising of its core temperature (Hammel 1968). Apparently, changing the temperature of as small an area as the hypothalamus is sufficient to "trick" the animal into initiating massive thermoregulatory adjustments. Hammel and his associates have shown that the response of an animal to hypothalamic heating or cooling is modified by the environmental temperature. For example, when the environmental temperature is 15°C, a dog's hypothalamus must be raised to over 41°C before it will begin to pant (a thermoregulatory effector response which leads to an increase in evaporative heat loss). At an environmental temperature of 30°C the dog will begin to pant when its hypothalamic temperature is raised to only 39.4°C (Figure 14) (Hellstrom and Hammel 1967). Data such as these have led to the theory that the regulation of body temperature is dependent upon neural inputs from thermal sensors in the skin as well as from thermal sensors in the hypothalamus.

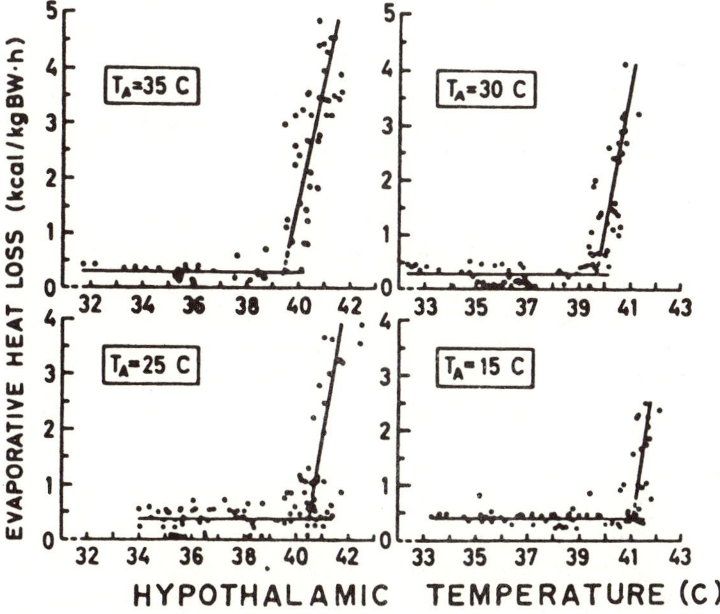

Figure 14. The relationship between hypothalamic temperatures and respiratory evaporative heat loss in a resting dog in four ambient temperatures. In a cool environment, the dog did not increase its evaporative heat loss (by panting) until its hypothalamic temperature had been raised to over 41°C. In a warm environment, panting began at a much lower hypothalamic temperature. (Based on Hellstrom and Hammel 1967.)

Within the past dozen years there have been numerous comparative studies concerned with the role of the hypothalamus in thermoregulation in the vertebrates. Thermodes have been placed into the hypothalamus of organisms from fishes through mammals and, with the possible exceptions of the big brown bat (*Eptesicus fuscus*) (Kluger and Heath 1971a) and the California quail (*Lophortyx californicus*) (Snapp et al. 1977), the hypothalamus has been found to be thermally sensitive (to varying degrees) in all these groups. In an endotherm like the house sparrow, warming the hypothalamus led to physiological and behavioral responses which reduced core temperature (Mills and Heath 1972a). Cooling the hypothalamus led to a rise in core temperature. In an ectotherm like the blue-tongued lizard, warming the rostral brainstem (an area surrounding the hypothalamus) made the lizard select a cooler environmental temperature. This resulted in a reduction in body temperature. Cooling the rostral brainstem led to the opposite results (Myhre and Hammel 1969). Again, peripheral inputs affected the responses to hypothalamic heating and cooling.

Based on these types of data, models of thermoregulation were developed which attempted to predict the thermal responses of a vertebrate based on inputs from the skin and the hypothalamus. The relative importance or "weighting" given to these two areas apparently varies depending upon what specific thermoregulatory response one is measuring, as well as upon the species being studied. These models, however, often fail to take into account information obtained over the last several years which has shown that internal or core areas other than the hypothalamus are also thermally sensitive, e.g. the spinal cord and the abdomen.

When the spinal cord of a dog is warmed, the dog reduces its core temperature; when the spinal cord is cooled, the dog raises its core temperature (Jessen and Mayer 1971). The magnitude of the response to heating or cooling the spinal cord is essentially the same as to heating or cooling the hypothalamus. Similar results have been obtained in vertebrates from amphibians (Duclaux et al. 1973), reptiles (Gorke et al. 1975), and birds (Rautenberg et al. 1972). In fact, in the pigeon, the importance of spinal cord temperature sensors appears to far outweigh that of the hypothalamic temperature sensors (Rautenberg et al. 1972). For an excellent review on the spinal cord's importance as a thermoregulatory sensor see Simon (1974).

When the abdomen of a sheep is warmed, the sheep initiates heat dissipating responses; when cooled, the sheep initiates the opposite responses (Rawson and Quick 1972)—convincing evidence that the abdominal viscera of these animals is thermally sensitive. Similar results have been reported for rabbits (Riedel et al. 1973) and cats (Hipskind and Hunter 1977). It is presently unknown whether abdominal temperature sensation is commonly found in the vertebrates.

Other areas are also thermally sensitive. For example, another central nervous area outside the hypothalamus and spinal cord that has been found to possess thermal sensitivity is the medulla oblongata (part of the hind brain) of cats (Chai and Wang 1970; Tabatabai 1972) and rats (Lipton 1973). Again, it is not presently known whether medullary temperature sensors are found in other groups of vertebrates. Clearly, any model of temperature regulation should incorporate those known extrahypothalamic deep body thermal receptors.

Table 1 summarizes our present understanding of the comparative aspects of thermal sensation in the vertebrates. The locations of temperature sensors throughout the vertebrates are remarkably conservative. The skin, the hypothalamus, the spinal cord, and perhaps other areas are

Table 1. Location of Thermally Sensitive Areas in the Vertebrates
(+ = area shown to be thermally sensitive; ? = area not yet investigated)

	Skin	*Hypothalamus*	*Spinal Cord*	*Abdomen*	*Other CNS Areas*
Mammals	+	+	+	+	+
Birds	+	+	+	?	?
Reptiles	+	+	+	?	?
Amphibians	+	+	+	?	?
Fishes	+	+	?	?	?

temperature sensitive in essentially all the vertebrates. Based on these similarities, it is obvious that the distinction between the endotherms (birds and mammals) and the ectotherms (most fishes, amphibians, and reptiles) is not on the sensory side of the thermoregulatory reflex (see Figure 11). We next turn our attention to the integration of body temperature—the second arm of this reflex.

Temperature Integration in the Vertebrates

In response to thermal stimuli, sensory or afferent information is carried by nerves to some area(s?) where this information is integrated. If the sensory information carries signals from a cold skin, spinal cord, hypothalamus, abdomen, etc., then the integration of these signals is conceptually relatively simple. Electrical (neural) and chemical (hormonal) signals leave the integrator(s?) and carry messages to the effectors to raise body temperature. Often these signals are conflicting. The core receptors could be sending signals that indicate that the animal's temperature is elevated (as during exercise) while the peripheral or skin receptors could be sending signals that indicate it is cold (as during exposure to low environmental temperatures). Now the role of the integrator(s?) is more complex. Little is known about how the integrator actually works. Most often the integration of almost any afferent signals (not only in the thermoregulatory system) is conceptualized as a black box with arrows entering (afferent signals) and others leaving (efferent signals). Our knowledge of the integration of body temperature is essentially at this low level of sophistication.

The location most commonly assigned to the integration of temperature is the hypothalamus. This area contains neurons which are sensitive to its own temperature as well as neurons which respond to the temperature of other thermally sensitive areas in the body. For example, activity in some neurons in the preoptic-anterior hypothalamus is increased when the skin (Hellon 1970), or spinal cord (Boulant and Hardy 1974) temperature is changed. The posterior hypothalamus also contains neurons which are responsive to thermal stimulation in other regions of the body such as the preoptic-anterior hypothalamus (Nutik 1973) and spinal cord (Wunnenberg and Hardy 1972). These types of data suggest that the hypothalamus might play a role in the integration of thermal information from other areas of the body.

Neuropharmacological data also suggest that the hypothalamus plays a key role in the integration of temperature. Nerves relay messages from one neuron to the next by releasing transmitter substances at a junction called the synapse. These chemicals are released from the presynaptic neuron, diffuse across the synaptic cleft to the postsynaptic neuron, and lead to either excitation or inhibition of the postsynaptic neuron. The unequivocal identification of specific neurotransmitters in the central nervous system has been difficult, although substances such as acetylcholine, norepinephrine, dopamine, histamine, gamma-aminobutyric acid (GABA), 5-hydroxytryptamine (5-HT, or serotonin), as well as a few others, are generally considered to be transmitters within the central nervous system. Of these, acetylcholine, norepinephrine, and 5-HT—and recently dopamine and histamine—have been thought to play a role in temperature regulation (Cox and Lomax 1977). If these neurotransmitters have a role in temperature regulation, then one might expect that an infusion of these substances into or near the hypothalamus could trigger some coordinated thermal response. The exogenous administration of these substances, however, has led to mixed results. For example, some investigators have reported that norepinephrine leads to a rise in body temperature and 5-HT leads to a fall in body temperature; others have reported the opposite results (see reviews in Bligh 1973; Hellon 1975). Similar mixed results have been reported for acetylcholine infusions. So, while these neurotransmitters might have some role in temperature regulation, it is presently unclear what that specific role might be.

Another group of substances which have received a great deal of attention lately are the prostaglandins (Figure 15). Prostaglandins are a group of ubiquitous lipid soluble com-

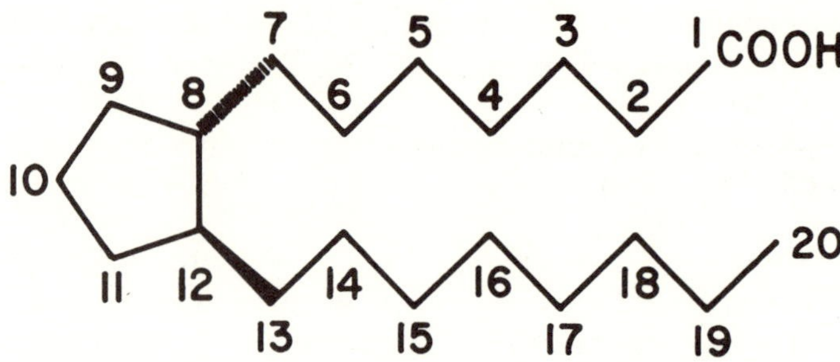

Figure 15. Basic structure of a prostaglandin. The different prostaglandins (E, F, A, etc.) are distinguished by the constituents of the cyclopentane ring. These main classes of prostaglandins are further subdivided in accord with the number of double bonds in the side chains. (Based on Douglas in Goodman and Gilman 1975.)

pounds which have been associated with just about every aspect of mammalian physiology. They have been studied for their effects on the cardiovascular system, gastrointestinal system, respiratory system, renal system, etc. (Douglas 1975). Naturally, thermal biologists have also investigated the effects of prostaglandins on temperature regulation. With few exceptions, intrahypothalamic injections of prostaglandins belonging to the E series have led to a rise in body temperature (Hellon 1975). As a result of this fairly consistent elevation in body temperature, and other aspects of prostaglandin pharmacology (to be described in detail in Chapter 2), prostaglandins have been implicated in the development of fever. It is unclear whether prostaglandins have any role in the normal regulation of body temperature.

Another interesting finding concerns the potential thermoregulatory role of sodium and calcium ions in the cerebrospinal fluid near or in the hypothalamus. When the ratio of these two ions is changed, one is able to predict the resultant changes in body temperature. For example, when the ratio of Na^+ to Ca^{++} is raised, body temperature becomes elevated; when it is lowered, body temperature falls (Myers and Veale 1970). In those species of mammals which have been studied, these results have usually been confirmed (Hellon 1975).

To summarize, infusions of putative neurotransmitters such as norepinephrine, 5-hydroxytryptamine, acetylcholine, and others, infusions of prostaglandins, and infusions of cations such as Ca^{++} and Na^{+} into the hypothalamus can lead to changes in body temperature. It is not known what, if any, physiological role these substances have under natural conditions. One major problem in almost all neuropharmacological studies is that the dose of drug necessary to elicit a response is generally far greater than would occur naturally. This is the case with the above studies. The problem is often rationalized away by the claim that these higher drug dosages are necessary since their specific receptors are not necessarily located near the sites of infusion. By the time these drugs have diffused to these receptors, they have been diluted and/or have been broken down or inactivated to some extent. This undoubtedly occurs in many cases; yet, it still makes the interpretation of the above data difficult. A second major problem with the results of pharmacological investigations into the central control of temperature regulation is that the results from different laboratories are so often contradictory. Broad interpretations or generalizations are therefore impossible.

Regardless of the specific role of these pharmacologic agents, they all tend to produce their greatest effects when injected into or near the hypothalamus. This could argue in favor of the hypothalamus having a key role in the integration of body temperature. Conversely, even if these drugs actually do have a physiological role in temperature regulation, an alternate interpretation could be that these results simply confirm earlier observations that the hypothalamus is one of the internal temperature sensors. These drugs might only be affecting these temperature sensors, without having any effect on the integration of body temperature.

A third type of experimental manipulation which has been used to implicate the hypothalamus as an integrator of thermal information is that of hypothalamic lesions. A lesion, as used in this context, refers to the ablation or removal of specific neural tissue. Lesions can be produced in specific areas of the brain by a variety of techniques. One of the more common ones involves passing current through a small wire which is insulated except for the tip. The wire is lowered into the brain of an anesthetized animal to the desired location based on a predetermined coordinate system. The tip is heated to temperatures above that which will destroy brain tissue, resulting in the abrupt removal of that area. By varying the length of time the current is passed, the diameter of the lesion-electrode, and the amount of current passed, the size of the lesion can be more or less adjusted. After a short recovery period of perhaps a few days to one week, one can compare the responses of the lesioned animal to that of a sham operated or control animal.

Lesions in the hypothalamus generally lead to varying degrees of deficits in the ability to thermoregulate. Generally, the animal can regulate its body temperature fairly well except when placed in extremely high or low environmental temperatures. Lesions in the anterior hypothalamus (and preoptic region) seldom eliminate all thermal responses, indicating that other areas are also contributing to the integration of body temperature (Kluger and Heath 1971b). Lesions in the posterior hypothalamus generally lead to more severe deficits in the regulation of body temperature (Ranson and Magoun 1939; Kluger et al. 1973b). Hypothalamic lesions have been shown to produce some degree of thermal impairment in mammals (Keller and McClaskey 1964), birds (Mills and Heath 1972b), reptiles (Kluger et al. 1973b; Berk and Heath 1976), and amphibians (Lillywhite 1971).

Once these experiments are completed, the animal is generally killed and its brain is sectioned and examined under the microscope for the location of the lesion. Even though one can accurately determine the location of the lesion, it is difficult to conclude with any degree of certainty whether that area is responsible for the produced deficit. It is often impossible to determine whether the deficit is attributable to the lesion having destroyed the area responsible for that response, or to the lesion having destroyed a neural pathway which passed through that area. With this as a cautionary note, one might still conclude that the results of lesion studies suggest that the hypothalamus has some role in temperature regulation. But, as in the neuropharmacological experiments, one cannot be certain, in many cases, whether the effects of the lesions are causing deficits in the sensing or integrating arms of the thermoregulatory reflex.

The results of hypothalamic electrical recordings during thermal stimulation of other areas of the body, hypothalamic infusions of pharmacological agents, and hypothalamic lesions all point toward the conclusion that the hypothalamus plays some role in the integration of body temperature in the vertebrates. Other areas, outside the hypothalamus, are probably also important in the integration of body temperature in vertebrates. Other areas, outside the hypothalamus, are probably also important in the integration of thermoregulatory reflexes (e.g. the medulla and the spinal cord). Fairly sophisticated models of temperature regulation, generally based on the hypothalamus as the sole integrator, have been described and are reviewed in some detail by Bligh (1973). These models are all theoretical and tend to underscore the fact that we know very little about how organisms actually integrate the thermal information from various regions of the body resulting in the regulation of body temperature.

One feature common to most of these models of thermoregulation is the concept of set-point (T_{set}), or its equivalent, to describe the regulated body temperature. The T_{set} is that temperature (or temperature range) around which the animal attempts to regulate its body temperature. When sensory inputs from the skin and core indicate that body temperature (T_b) is greater than T_{set}, the animal initiates effector responses which lower T_b. When $T_b < T_{set}$, these effector responses tend to raise T_b toward the set-point temperature. The set-point temperature is, of course, not a constant, T_{set} being lowered during sleep, anesthesia, hibernation, etc. and raised during infections resulting in fever. Almost all vertebrates from fishes to mammals behave as though they regulated their body temperatures around some set-point or set-range (perhaps with a high set-point at the upper limit and a low set-point at the lower limit of the range) (Heath 1968). Clearly, the concept of a set-point is important for conceptualizing the process of thermoregulatory integration.

Temperature Effectors in the Vertebrates

The effectors represent the third arm of the thermoregulatory reflex (see Figure 11). Information from the temperature sensors is fed into the integrator(s?), and when $T_{set} \neq T_b$ the net effect is the activation of thermoregulatory effector responses. These responses might involve physiological or behavioral alterations by the organism and can lead to changes in the organism's rate of heat loss, heat gain, and heat production.

Recall that heat can be exchanged between an organism and its environment by conduction, convection, radiation, and evaporation (see Figure 4). The effector responses available to a thermoregulator take advantage of these physical laws of heat exchange to minimize or maximize energy exchange. The rate of heat lost by an animal to its environment can be increased or decreased by altering any one (or more) of these four modes of heat exchange. Heat can also be gained from the environment by the three modes of dry heat exchange—conduction, convection, and radiation. Heat is produced internally as a result of an organism's metabolic processes. Basically, then, the thermoregulator maintains a relatively constant body temperature by physiological and behavioral adjustments which utilize the four modes of energy exchange between an organism and its environment and by modulating its rate of internal heat production. The general thermoregulatory effector responses available to vertebrates are often divided into four general catagories: (1) changes in metabolic heat production; (2) changes in skin blood flow; (3) changes in evaporative water loss; and (4) a variety of behavioral responses. These specific effector responses are described below.

1. Changes in Metabolic Heat Production. The sum of an organism's biochemical reactions is its metabolism. These biochemical reactions ultimately result in the generation of heat. The amount of heat an organism generates is propor-

tional to the rates of these reactions and is often referred to as its metabolic rate or metabolic heat production. An endotherm which is at rest in a neutral environment and is post absorptive (not absorbing food from the digestive tract) has a minimal metabolic heat production known as its "basal metabolic rate" (BMR). To maintain a constant body temperature in a cold environment, the endotherm can increase its metabolic rate above this BMR and thus generate extra heat. There are, naturally, limits to the magnitude of this increase in an organism's metabolic activities, although a doubling or tripling of the metabolic heat production in response to exposure to the cold is not uncommon.

The increase in metabolic heat occurs by increased skeletal muscle activity (often as shivering) or by the breakdown (catabolism) of fat. This latter process occurs without any visible body movement and is referred to as nonshivering thermogenesis (NST). Shivering is essentially the repeated synchronous contractions of both the flexor and extensor skeletal muscles (Bligh 1973). As a result of this increase in internal work, without any external work, a large amount of heat is liberated. Shivering is initiated upon exposure to the cold, most often triggered by cooling the peripheral thermoreceptors. Under certain natural and experimental conditions, shivering can also be stimulated by cooling the deep body thermoreceptors. Although the activation of these skeletal muscles is via somatic efferent nerves, shivering is generally an involuntary response to cold exposure. Birds and mammals are known to shiver as a thermoregulatory adjustment to the cold. In reptiles, pythons apparently shiver during the incubation of their eggs and thus maintain a temperature several degrees Celsius above the environmental temperature (Hutchison et al. 1966). Although it is not considered shivering, several species of large, fast-swimming fishes such as the mako and porbeagle sharks (Carey and Teal 1969) and the bluefin tuna (Carey and Lawson 1973) also generate sufficient heat in their skeletal muscles to maintain a body temperature more than 5°C above the water temperature. There has even been a great deal of speculation that dinosaurs and related extinct reptiles were endothermic, and as a result would have undoubtedly shivered to maintain their body temperature upon exposure to the cold (Desmond 1975).

Nonshivering thermogenesis is the other means by which endotherms generate significant amounts of heat above the basal metabolic heat production. NST is basically due to the oxidation of fat within adipose tissue and results in the production of a great deal of heat. The specific biochemical processes involved in NST are unknown. Generally, NST is attributed to a special type of fat called brown fat. Brown fat, however, is probably not a prerequisite for NST since young birds, which apparently do not possess brown fat, are also thought to be capable of NST (Freeman 1966; Wekstein and Zolman 1968). Brown fat is most often found in young mammals, and in older small mammals such as rodents and bats which have been exposed to the cold for lengthy periods (cold acclimated). The fat itself is not actually brown, but is yellow in color; the brown coloration of brown fat is due to the heavy vascularization of this tissue as well as to the high content of respiratory pigments within the fat (Hull 1971). Exposure to the cold, either external or internal, can trigger the catabolism of this tissue with the resultant release of heat. Norepinephrine released from sympathetic nerves to the brown fat, and to a lesser extent from the adrenal medulla, triggers its oxidation (Jansky 1973). In some animals, hibernating bats for example, virtually all of the heat produced during their arousal from hiberation is attributable to norepinephrine-induced NST (Figure 16).

Thus, whereas mammals and birds are capable of generating significant amounts of heat by NST, the ability to generate significant amounts of heat above the BMR by skeletal muscular activity is not a characteristic belonging solely to them. Some species of fishes and reptiles (both living and extinct?) as well as some organisms belonging to other phyla, such as certain species of insects, can also generate enough heat to be considered endotherms. As we will see later, the primary distinction between the endotherms and the ectotherms with regard to the regulation of body temperature (including the sensing, integrating, and effecting limbs of

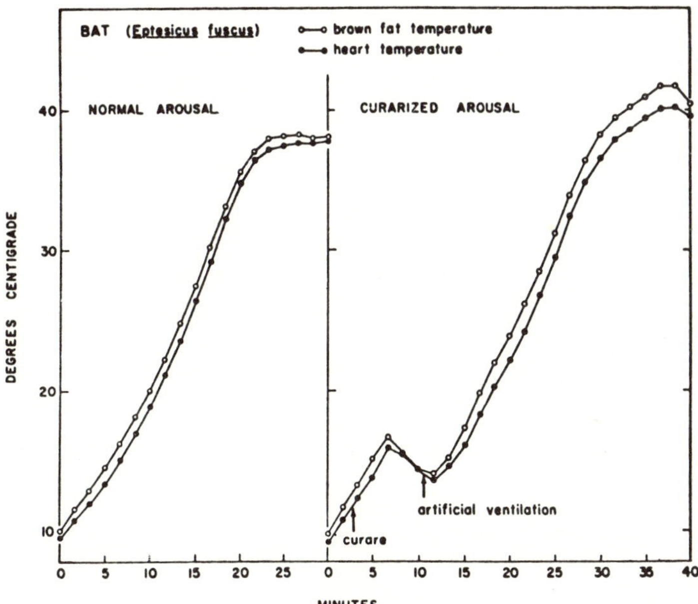

Figure 16. Comparison of the rate of arousal from hibernation in a normal and curarized bat. Curare is an effective inhibitor of skeletal muscle contraction. As a result, virtually all the heat produced by a curarized animal must come from nonshivering thermogenesis. In both the normal and curarized bat, the brown fat temperature was consistently around 1°C above the heart temperature. It is clear from this figure that most of the heat produced by the arousing bat comes from NST. (From Hayward and Lyman 1967.)

the reflex) is the ability of endotherms to produce substantial amounts of heat by shivering or nonshivering means.

2. Changes in Skin Bood Flow. The rate of heat exchange between an organism and its environment can be affected by adjusting the amount of blood flowing to the skin. These vasomotor changes can result in increased or decreased blood flow to an area. Increased blood flow is generally caused by vasodilation of the arterioles leading to that vascular bed or tissue. Vasodilation, an increase in the radius of the arterioles, can lead to enormous increases in blood flow

to a region (flow is proportional to the radius of a tube raised to the fourth power). For example, a vasodilated area of skin often receives 100 times the blood flow compared to the area when it is vasoconstricted (Rowell 1974).

The control over vasomotor responses to the skin is thought to be via sympathetic nerves as well as by local, or intrinsic, mechanisms. The warming of various core thermal receptors leads to reflex peripheral vasodilation. Cooling results in peripheral vasoconstriction. Local heating of the skin also induces vasodilation; mild cooling, again, has the opposite effect.

Because blood has such a high specific heat (close to that of water), changes in the regional distribution of blood can result in large changes in an organism's body temperature. The manner in which changes in the distribution of blood flow can play an important role in thermoregulation is illustrated by the following example. When an endotherm, such as the laboratory rabbit, is in an environment which is thermally neutral or even slightly cool, say 10°C, its skin temperature will be fairly low. This indicates that it is peripherally vasoconstricted. Its large, poorly insulated ears, for example, will be only a few degrees above the environmental temperature. The rabbit has shunted blood from its periphery to its core. It has, in effect, sacrificed its peripheral temperature (shell) to maintain a warm and constant core temperature (ca. 39°C in the rabbit). The periphery now serves as an effective insulative barrier against the cold. Since ear skin temperature is only about 4°C higher than the environmental temperature, the amount of heat transferred from the vasoconstricted ears to its surroundings by conduction, convection, and radiation will be small compared to what happens when the ears are vasodilated. During exercise leading to a rise in core temperature, skin blood flow increases, resulting in a rise in skin temperature. The shell has essentially disappeared as warm blood is carried to the skin where conductive, convective, and radiative heat exchange carries substantial amounts of heat away from the body. This increase in the gradient between ear and environmental temperature results in approximately a ninefold increase in heat loss from the ears (Figure 17).

Changes in skin blood flow in response to thermal stimuli have been described for mammals, birds, and recently for reptiles. In birds and mammals, vasodilation generally leads to an increase in heat loss, the exception being when skin temperature is less than environmental temperature. Vasoconstriction of skin blood vessels generally leads to a decrease in heat loss—again, the exception being when skin temperature is less than environmental temperature.

In ectothermic reptiles, peripheral vasomotion tends to

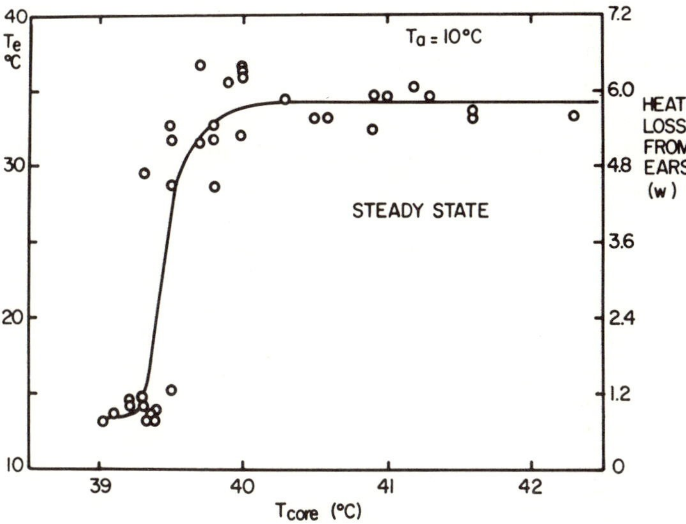

Figure 17. Ear temperature (T_e) and heat loss (in watts) at different levels of core temperature in New Zealand white rabbits in an environmental temperature of 10°C. Core temperature was raised above resting values (ca. 39.3°C) by forcing the rabbits to run on a treadwheel. Above a core temperature of about 39.5°C, ear blood flow increased, resulting in an increase in ear temperature. Based on earlier studies, we were able to calculate the amount of heat lost from the ears at different ear-environmental gradients. In these experiments, ear vasodilation resulted in an increase in heat loss of approximately 5 watts. (From Kluger et al. 1973a.)

have a somewhat different effect from that found in birds and mammals. Recall that ectotherms rely on external sources of heat to raise their body temperature to their "active" or "preferred" temperature. Cowles (1958), in a fascinating paper concerned with the origins of peripheral vasomotor control, was probably the first to suggest that reptiles have some control over their skin blood flow and that this could be an important thermoregulatory effector response. This has subsequently been confirmed in numerous studies in which blood flow has actually been measured (White 1976). Warming the skin results in peripheral vasodilation. This warm blood is then carried back to the reptile's core and results in an increased rate of temperature rise in warming reptiles. When the warm thermal stimulus is removed from the skin, the skin becomes peripherally vasoconstricted. Body temperature now falls; but, since the "shell" is peripherally vasoconstricted, this decline in body temperature is slower than would have occurred had the skin remained peripherally vasodilated. By becoming peripherally vasodilated in the heat, and peripherally vasoconstricted in the cold, these ectotherms are able to maintain their body temperature in their preferred range for greater periods of time.

So we see that in both endotherms and ectotherms, peripheral vasoconstriction usually decreases heat loss. However, whereas peripheral vasodilation generally increases heat loss in endotherms, this response generally leads to an increase in heat gain in ectotherms.

3. Changes in Evaporative Water Loss. The third thermoregulatory effector response available to animals is that of increasing or decreasing evaporative water loss. The evaporation of water can result in substantial cooling; however, for water to evaporate, there must be some difference in vapor pressure between the organism and its environment. This clearly precludes evaporation of water as an effective thermoregulatory mechanism in aquatic vertebrates. Terrestrial vertebrates lose water by two avenues—the respiratory tract and the skin. When the relative humidity is less than 100%, water loss from the respiratory tract and skin is

inevitable. Air which is expired from the respiratory tract is generally considered to be close to fully saturated with water (McCutchan and Taylor 1951; Schmidt-Nielsen 1972). The rate of evaporative heat loss increases linearly as the difference in vapor pressure between the inspired air and the expired air increases. Many terrestrial vertebrates have some control over the amount of this respiratory evaporative water (heat) loss. Evaporation from the respiratory tract can be increased by increasing the volume of air breathed per unit time, a phenomenon known as panting.

Panting has been found to be a thermoregulatory response in mammals, birds, and reptiles and is triggered by an elevation in either deep body or peripheral temperature (Richards 1970; Crawford and Barber 1974). Although the process of panting leads to an elevation in the metabolic heat produced by an animal, the magnitude of the respiratory evaporative heat loss is generally sufficiently great to make panting a significant avenue of heat loss.

The other physiological means by which organisms lose heat by evaporation of water is via the skin. All terrestrial organisms lose some water through the skin by simple diffusional processes. As this is not a regulated process, it is not considered to be a thermoregulatory effector mechanism. An animal can facilitate evaporative water loss from the skin by such behavioral means as licking its skin (or fur or feathers), urinating on itself, wallowing in mud or water, etc. These behavioral effector responses will be discussed later. Another way evaporation of water from the skin is facilitated is by sweating.

Sweating, as a thermoregulatory response, is known to occur only in mammals. Sweating occurs from specialized glands located in the dermal layers of the skin and is initiated by thermal stimulation of either the core or peripheral thermal receptors (Nadel et al. 1971). In certain animals (e.g. kangaroos, horses, goats) the control of these sweat glands is considered to be virtually entirely under the influence of adrenergic neurons (those that release the catecholamines, norepinephrine and epinephrine) (Bligh 1973; Dawson et al. 1974). In others (e.g. human beings, cats, rats) sweating is thought to be under the control of cholinergic neurons (those that release acetylcholine) (Bligh 1973). There is, however, some evidence that catecholamines also play some role in sweating in human beings (Allen and Roddie 1972).

Loss of heat via sweating can be enormous, particularly in such highly specialized organisms as human beings. With our nearly naked skin, we can easily lose more than 1 liter of sweat per hour. A loss of 1 liter of sweat results in about 580 Kcal of heat being dissipated, about six times the resting metabolic heat production of most people.

4. Behavioral Effector Responses. As briefly mentioned above, one effective behavioral response available to terrestrial vertebrates employs the evaporation of water. Turtles, for example, when heat stressed, will salivate and then proceed to smear the saliva onto their front legs. Turtles will also urinate and spread the urine on their rear legs (Riedesel et al. 1971). Horned lizards lose heat by the evaporation of cloacal fluids from their body (Heath 1965). Some birds, such as storks and vultures, when heat stressed, also urinate on themselves, resulting in substantial cooling (Bartholomew 1977). In mammals, behavioral cooling using evaporation of liquids takes many forms. In some mammals, such as rats and bats, spreading of saliva is observed during exposure to high environmental temperatures (Stricker and Hainsworth 1970; Kluger and Heath 1971b). Bats have also been observed to urinate on themselves in response to heat stress. Many of the larger mammals tend to wallow in mud (pigs) or in shallow water (elephants, people) as a thermoregulatory response to the heat.

All vertebrates rely on some locomotor behavior to regulate their body temperature. These changes might involve gross movements or more subtle postural changes leading to increases or decreases in the rate of energy exchange between the organism and its environment. Fishes will, for example, if given a choice of environmental temperatures, select a "preferred" body temperature (see, for example, Reynolds et al. 1976). (The knowledge of the "preferred" temperature of certain species of fishes has been used with varying degrees of success by fishermen.) Amphibians also have "preferred" temperature ranges, although in many cases these ranges can be fairly broad (20°C or more) (Brattstrom 1970). Bullfrogs, however, select a body temperature within a fairly narrow range (26°-33°C) (Lillywhite 1970). When their body temperature goes above or below this range, they will change their microclimate or body postures, resulting in the return to this temperature range. Reptiles largely rely on postural and/or locomotor changes for much of their thermoregulation. Many reptiles will bask in the early morning until their body temperatures rise to levels near their "preferred" range. Once within this range, which varies from one species to the next, the reptile will often shuttle between the shade and sunlight to maintain its temperature within this range. Often, a subtle postural change, such as changing its angle of orientation toward the sunlight, is sufficient to allow the animal to remain active without retreating to a cooler area such as its burrow or to a tree (Heath 1965). Endotherms also use similar types of behavioral responses to thermoregulate. In the cold, birds have often been observed to orient themselves toward the sunlight, and in the heat they often have been observed to retreat to cooler shaded areas (Dawson and Hudson 1970). Mammals also employ these behavioral responses. We are all no doubt aware of some of the behavioral responses of dogs and cats to the heat and cold. During the winter, one often can observe these animals basking in the sunlight by a closed window or near a warm radiator. In the summer, they will often be found in a cool damp area beneath a tree, porch, etc. These types of behavioral responses are fairly characteristic of most mammals.

Endotherms such as birds and mammals also rely on changes in insulation to assist in their regulation of body temperature. Birds are known to fluff their feathers and to huddle when cold (Dawson and Hudson 1970). Mammals will employ similar insulative responses in the cold (e.g. by piloerecting their fur, and by decreasing the surface area exposed to the cold by huddling). In response to long-term exposure to the cold, some mammals are known to undergo a thickening of the fur resulting in an improvement of their insulation (Webster 1974).

Although one often thinks of ectotherms as relying on behavioral means, and of endotherms as relying on physiological means to regulate their body temperatures, this is clearly not the case. Both groups rely on a host of physiological and behavioral responses to arrive at their regulated body temperatures. In fact, most of the regulation of body temperature in endotherms such as ourselves is accomplished by behavior.

A persons' metabolic heat production in a neutral environmental temperature of about 30°C might be 70 Kcal/hr. Without relying on behavioral thermoregulatory responses, when the environmental temperature is reduced to 0°C, the metabolic heat production would probably rise to over 110 Kcal/hr (Grollman 1930). The increase in metabolic heat production would be the result of intense shivering and other muscular movements. This thermoregulatory effector response, however, is almost always prevented in human beings by behavioral thermoregulatory responses. In the cold, we wear warmer clothing and drink hot liquids. We also behaviorally thermoregulate by avoiding the cold. We build homes heated to about 20°C and even attempt to maintain our cars at this temperature. Behavioral thermoregulation in response to the cold saves us this large expenditure of energy.

In a warm environment of, for example 40°C, we would evaporate large amounts of water in order to maintain our body temperature at about 37°C. Again, this expenditure of energy (and fluids) is generally avoided, or at least moderated, by behavioral thermoregulatory responses. We reduce our insulation by removing clothing, cool ourselves by drinking cold fluids and spreading cool water on our body surface, and generally tend to avoid the heat by moving into the shade of trees, our cooler homes, etc. Basically we rely on thermoregulatory behavioral responses to reduce the need for the physiological effector responses of increasing heat production in the cold and increasing body fluid losses in the heat.

Summary

From this short introduction to the various components of the thermoregulatory reflex arc, we can see that the fundamental difference between endotherms and ectotherms lies not in the sensory or integrating arms of this reflex, but rather in the effector arm. We have seen that both groups have peripheral thermoreceptors located in the skin, and core thermoreceptors located in the hypothalamus, spinal cord, and probably elsewhere. The integration of the thermal information is thought to reside in the hypothalamus and in other central nervous sites, although this is still not adequately understood. The primary distinction between ectotherms and endotherms resides in the effector limb; it is not that endotherms utilize physiological effector mechanisms whereas ectotherms utilize behavioral ones, but rather, that endotherms have the metabolic machinery to generate sufficient amounts of internal heat to raise their core temperature. This ability to produce large amounts of heat, furthermore, is not a characteristic unique to birds and mammals. Examples of endothermy can be found in fishes and reptiles (as well as in plants and insects). Thus, it is basically this one component of the effector limb of the thermoregulatory reflex that distinguishes the endotherms from the ectotherms.

The reader may wonder why I have devoted so much space to essentially an introductory chapter in a text on the evolution and adaptive value of fever. Fever, as we shall see in Chapter 2, is thought to result from a resetting of the hypothalamic and other central nervous area thermostats, altering, in some way, either the thermally sensitive and/or integrative neurons. Since these two limbs of the thermoregulatory reflex are phylogenetically conservative (that is, similar in all the vertebrate classes), we suspected that the ability to develop a fever might also be found in such nonmammalian classes as the endothermic birds and the ectothermic reptiles, amphibians, and fishes. If we could demonstrate this long phylogenetic history for fever, we thought (for reasons I will explain in some detail in Chapter

4) that we would now have a more suitable animal model than the commonly used laboratory rabbit to investigate various aspects of fever and its role in disease. But, before I can describe the investigations into the evolution and adaptive value of fever, it is first necessary to have a fundamental understanding of the basic biology of fever, the subject of Chapter 2.

2. The Biology of Fever

Historical Observations

A relationship between fever and disease was apparent even to Hippocrates some 2,400 years ago. He recognized fever to be an important symptom of illness (Coxe 1846). Fever was also observed following various types of injuries. Hippocrates noted that inflammation, whether it resulted from injuries or from unknown causes, was often associated with fever. His writings are also filled with somewhat cryptic phrases alluding to his belief that fever was often a healthy sign during an infection; that is, that fever might play a beneficial role.

Hippocrates, of course, was on shaky ground when he attempted to explain the actual causes of fever. According to Hippocrates, fever was related, in some manner, to the separation in the body of cold and heat (Jones 1923). When these "powers" were mixed, a person was healthy; but when they became entirely separated, the person was in pain and apparently developed a fever (Duran-Reynals 1946). In the case of malarial fever, this process was related to the four humors (blood, phlegm, yellow bile, and black bile), with bile being the most important.

While it is undoubtedly true that much of Hippocrates' writings concerning fever have little scientific basis, it is nevertheless remarkable that he was in many cases able to make accurate statements concerning the biology of fever and disease. Unavailable to Hippocrates were even the crudest instruments (by today's standards) necessary to investigate this area. One of the most important, and fundamental, to current investigators is some form of instrument to measure temperature. Major advances in the understanding of the relationship between fever and disease had to await the development of the thermometer some 2,000 years after Hippocrates' death.

Thermometry has had an interesting history. While it was shown by Hero of Alexandria that air expands on heating and contracts on cooling, it was not until about 1,750 years later that an actual thermometer was invented. According to historians of science, until the 1600s there existed no apparatus for measuring temperature. (It was not until the middle 1700s that the distinction between temperature and heat was clarified [Marantz 1969].)

Without a temperature measuring device of some sort, it is virtually impossible to investigate fever carefully. For example, while it is often claimed that by feeling one's forehead one can ascertain whether one is febrile or afebrile, this is highly unreliable. A person can have an afebrile body temperature, and if peripherally vasodilated (for whatever reason) will appear to have a fever by the above method. The converse is also true. Therefore, an instrument was needed which could measure the temperature of deep body tissues.

It is unclear who actually deserves the credit for the invention of the thermometer. According to Bolton (1900), Galileo should be given credit for this invention, although Taylor (1942) suggests that others, perhaps Sanctorius, may have preceded Galileo. Both Galileo, the famed physicist and astronomer, and Sanctorius, considered by some to be the first physiologist, worked at Padua at roughly the same time. According to Bolton, Galileo invented (or reinvented) the thermometer in 1592 and used this invention in his public lectures. This thermometer consisted of an inverted glass bulb, connected to a long tube. The tube was placed in a reservoir and filled partially with either water or wine (Figure 18). In one of Galileo's letters, he says: "when the air in the bulb contracts through cold, the wine in the stem rises to take the place of the void thus formed, and when the air is warmed it is rarefied and takes up more space so that it drives out and presses down the wine; from this it follows that cold is nothing but absence of heat" (Bolton 1900). Since the reservoir was open to the air, this thermometer was actually an air thermoscope and as such also measured changes in barometric pressure. Sealed thermometers, de-

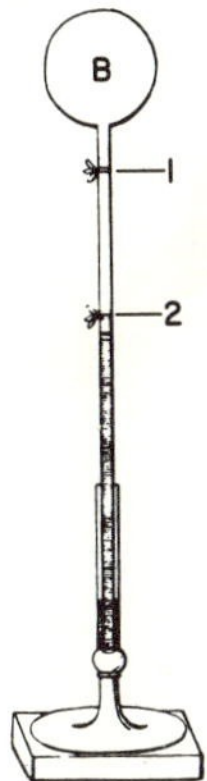

Figure 18. Sanctorius' thermometer, similar to the one described by Galileo. When the air in the bulb (B) was warmed, the fluid in the stem fell from point 1 to point 2. Note that the reservoir was open to the air in these early thermometers.

pending on the expansion of liquids and independent of barometric pressure, were not made until about fifty years later (Bolton 1900). Galileo's thermometer was apparently marked out in degrees and was used to measure the relative temperatures of different environments on a daily and seasonal basis.

The first published accounts of the thermometer, however, appeared in the writings of Sanctorius in 1611 (Taylor 1942). Sanctorius had already applied this instrument to his physiological investigations. In later works, Sanctorius described the use of the thermometer in his studies on the normal and febrile temperatures of people (Figure 19). This instrument was used to determine the "heat" of a patient by measuring his oral temperature. The rate of fall of the liquid in the thermometer during ten beats of a pulsilogium (small pendulum used to measure time) was compared in healthy and sick people. During disease, the rate of fall in the liquid was faster, indicating a higher temperature or fever (Taylor 1942). Sanctorius wrote: "Using that instrument, one can also make a comparison of the warmth—and particularly the heat of fever—from one day to another, or

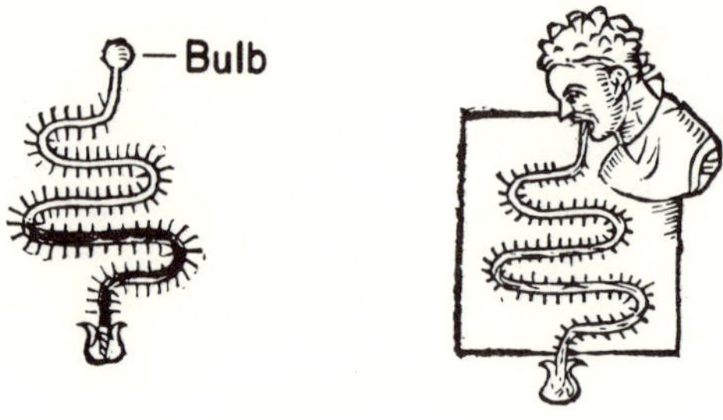

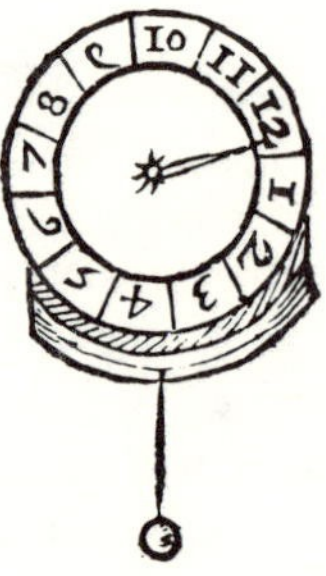

Figure 19. Reproduction of Sanctorius' drawings of the use of his thermometer for measuring the temperature of patients. The bulb was placed into the mouth of a patient and the rate of fall of the fluid was used to indicate whether the patient had a fever. Notice that the thermometer was marked off in equal gradations and that a small pendulum was used to record time.

from one paroxysm to another; from there we put together with certainty, whether the heat of fever increases or decreases, and by how many degrees" (Benzinger 1977). Sanctorius was thus perhaps the first to recognize that a person has a normal body temperature during health and that variations in body temperature during disease could be used as an indicator of the status of the infection (Bolton 1900).

A sidenote to the early history of thermometry concerns the use of reliable scales. In the late 1600s it was suggested by Renaldini that the melting point of ice and the boiling point of water be used as two fixed points on a thermometer

(Bolton 1900). Shortly thereafter, Farenheit suggested a series of gradations based on the three fixed points of 0° as the temperature of a mixture of ice, water, and salt, 32° as the temperature of ice and water without the salt, and 96° as a person's oral temperature. "If however," Farenheit writes, "the temperature of a person suffering from fever . . . is to be taken, another thermometer must be used having a scale lengthened to 128 to 132°. . . ; I do not think . . . that the degrees named will ever be exceeded in any fever" (Bolton 1900).

Somewhat later, the centigrade scale was developed. Although this scale is usually attributed to Anders Celsius, this is not entirely accurate. For some reason—perhaps related to the fact that in earlier thermometers the fluid level fell when the temperature of the bulb was elevated and rose when the temperature of the bulb was depressed—Celsius' scale had the freezing point of water at 100° and the boiling point at 0°. It is currently thought that this scale was inverted to its present form (0°C = f.p. of water, and 100°C = b.p. of water) by Pierre Martel in 1742 (Bryden 1971), and it may be that the centigrade scale should be gradated in degrees "Martel" rather than in degrees "Celsius" (see Pirie 1972).

Thus, since the middle 1700s an instrument has been available for the accurate recording of body temperature during periods of health and disease. Not long after the development of the germ theory of disease in the middle 1800s, experiments were being performed which attempted to demonstrate the relationship between fever and inflammation in experimental animals (see Bennett and Beeson's review 1950). Some of these early experiments will be described later.

By the 1870s, the monitoring of body temperature had become an important diagnostic tool. Wunderlich was extremely instrumental in establishing the practice of accurately monitoring and recording the body temperatures of patients. In his book, *Medical Thermometry* (1871), he described the value of the thermometer in medical practice, claiming that "the use of the thermometer in disease is, therefore, an objective, physical method of investigation, which gives exact and accurate results, in signs which can be measured and expressed numerically; which is delicate enough to follow every step of the changing processes of the organism, and places at the disposal of the practitioner a phenomenon dependent upon the sum total of the organic changes in the body." Wunderlich carefully recorded the body temperatures of healthy and ill patients and established that temperatures below 38°C were probably normal and those above probably febrile. Among his many observations, he noted that children tend to respond to infection with greater fevers than those found in adults, and that old people often have a depressed febrile response. He also described, and presented as graphs, the patterns of the febrile responses in numerous diseases. Wunderlich's convincing arguments for the monitoring of body temperature as an invaluable aid to the physician in both the diagnosis and treatment of various diseases initiated the modern practice of systematically recording the body temperature of hospitalized patients.

Set-Point Concept and Fever

The exact nature of fever was, however, still unknown. In fact, an acceptable definition of "fever" was not made until the 1870s when Liebermeister suggested that fever is not the result of an inability of the organism to regulate body temperature, but rather that the organism is simply regulating its body temperature at a higher level (Liebermeister 1887). This view that fever was a regulated higher body temperature was based on Liebermeister's experimental observations that the body temperature of a febrile subject returned to its previously raised level after warming or cooling of the body (Snell and Atkins 1968). Liebermeister differentiated between passive rises in body temperature, as might occur during exposure to a hot environment or during heavy physical work, and fever. In fever, the person's heat production became elevated, while at the same time, the individual's heat loss decreased (Liebermeister 1887).

Much evidence has accumulated which supports Liebermeister's definition of fever. Fever is currently defined by using the helpful concept of set-point. Snell and Atkins (1968), for example, have defined four categories of body temperature based on the set-point theory of temperature regulation. Their classification scheme is as follows:

1. Normothermia—where set-point and actual body temperature are essentially the same (occurs most of the time).
2. Hypothermia—where set-point may or may not be normal but actual body temperature is below this set-point (can occur in response to disease, drugs, or cold exposure).
3. Hyperthermia—where set-point may or may not be normal but actual body temperature is higher than this set-point (can occur in response to disease, drugs, or heat exposure).
4. Fever—where set-point is raised and deep body temperature may or may not be raised to the same level.

We see that their definition of fever, using the modern lexicon, is essentially the same as Liebermeister's.

Bligh (1973) has diagrammed these various states of body temperature by showing the changes in set-point and the resultant body temperature as an individual goes from normothermia to fever and back again to normothermia (Figure 20). At time A, body temperature (T_b) is approximately equal to set-point temperature (T_{set}). In response to some infection, the T_{set} is raised and the individual has a fever (time B). Since T_b is less than T_{set}, the individual is hypothermic. As such, all the effector mechanisms which will elevate body temperature are initiated. For example, the individual increases its metabolic heat production, decreases its heat loss by decreasing skin blood flow and evaporative heat loss, and also employs behavioral responses which lead to a raised T_b. In the case of human beings, these behavioral responses may include raising room temperature, drinking hot liquids, putting on warmer clothing or blankets, and postural changes which decrease heat loss. Once $T_b = T_{set}$ (time C) the individual is once again normothermic; yet he

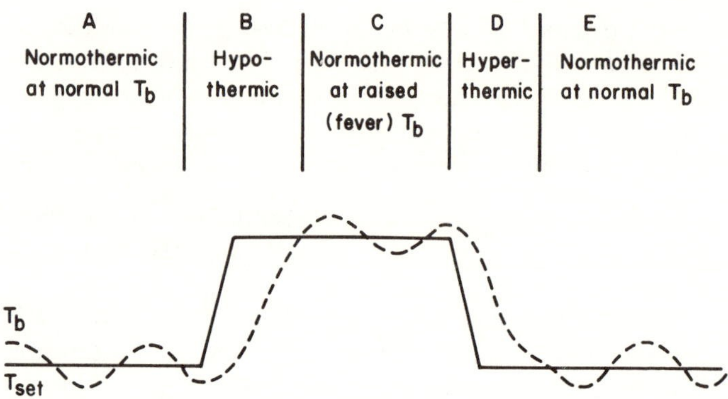

Figure 20. A diagrammatic representation of the relation between core temperature (T_b) and the set-point temperature (T_{set}); A) before the onset of fever; B) during the rising phase of fever; C) during maintained fever; D) during the subsiding phase; and E) after the return to normal thermoregulation. (From Bligh 1973.)

still is febrile. When the fever "breaks," T_{set} returns to its original level; however, T_b is now considerably above T_{set} (time D). The individual is now hyperthermic and as such initiates those responses, familiar to all of us, which lead to a reduction in body temperature. There is an increase in blood flow to the skin, an increase in evaporative heat loss (sweating), a reduction in metabolic heat production, and again, many behavioral responses such as lowering room temperature, drinking cold liquids, etc. When $T_b = T_{set}$ (time E) the individual is once again normothermic.

There have been two types of studies which have been used to support the "elevated set-point" theory of fever. The first involves the physiological and behavioral responses of the intact organism. For example, Cooper et al. (1964) found that during fever in man, thermoregulatory responses were still functional. The primary difference between febrile and afebrile subjects was that during the rising phase of fever, the response to an external heat load was diminished or absent. In this study they immersed the arms of subjects in warm water. This led to vasodilation in a febrile or febrile subjects (when $T_b = T_{set}$); but, during the rising phase of fever (when $T_b < {}_{set}$) this heat load had little effect on skin blood flow.

Cabanac and his associates have shown experimentally that during a fever, mammals will employ behavioral responses in order to elevate their body temperature. In one study, dogs were placed in a temperature controlled chamber where they could behaviorally adjust the amount of cool or warm air being blown into the chamber. When febrile, the dogs responded by increasing the amount of warm air and decreasing the amount of cool air entering the chamber (Cabanac et al. 1970). In a study involving human subjects, Cabanac and Massonnet (1974) found similar results. Human beings were sitting in a constant temperature bath (at 30° or 40°C). The subject's left arm and hand were outside the bath and that hand was placed in a glove which was capable of being heated to between 10° and 50°C. Each subject could adjust the temperature of the glove. During a fever, the subjects selected a warmer hand temperature. As their core temperature became raised, each subject (whether febrile or afebrile) selected a cooler glove temperature. However, in febrile subjects this response occurred at a higher body temperature, supporting the theory that the set-point for the regulation of body temperature had been elevated (Figure 21).

Similar results have been found during warming of specific internal thermal sensors such as the hypothalamus. For example, Sharp and Hammel (1972) have shown that warming the hypothalamus of dogs leads to increased salivation. During fever, the hypothalamic temperature must be raised to a higher level before salivation would begin.

Studies on nonmammalian vertebrates have shown that in ectotherms, such as the desert iguana, fever results in their selection of a warmer microenvironment (Vaughn et al. 1974). Lizards were placed in a chamber in which one end was heated to approximately 50°C and the other to approximately 30°C. To regulate their body temperature at their preferred temperature of around 38°C, the lizards shuttled between these two temperature extremes (Figure 22). Resting on either side for too long led to body tempera-

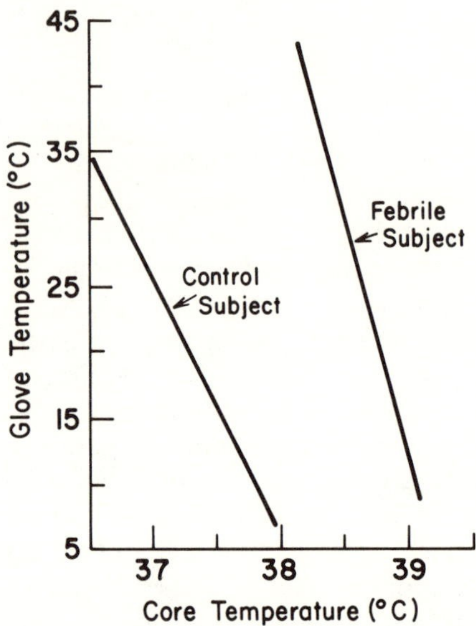

Figure 21. Preferred glove temperature vs. core temperature in human beings. Each subject sat in a warm bath (40°C). As core (esophageal) temperature rose, each subject selected a cooler glove (hand) temperature. Note that when the subject was made febrile, a higher body temperature was reached before he selected a cooler glove temperature. These data are in agreement with the raised set-point theory of fever. (Redrawn from Cabanac and Massonnet 1974.)

tures considerably above or below 38°C. During infection, the lizards developed a fever, resulting in their spending greater lengths of time on the warm side of the chamber. As a result, body temperature rose to approximately 41°C. This is a clear demonstration of the regulation of body temperature at a raised level during fever. Similar results have been reported in other classes of vertebrates and will be described in detail in Chapter 3.

The theory that during fever the organism's set-point is elevated has also received support from neurophysiological data. If one assumes that the thermally sensitive neurons found in the hypothalamus have some role in thermoregula-

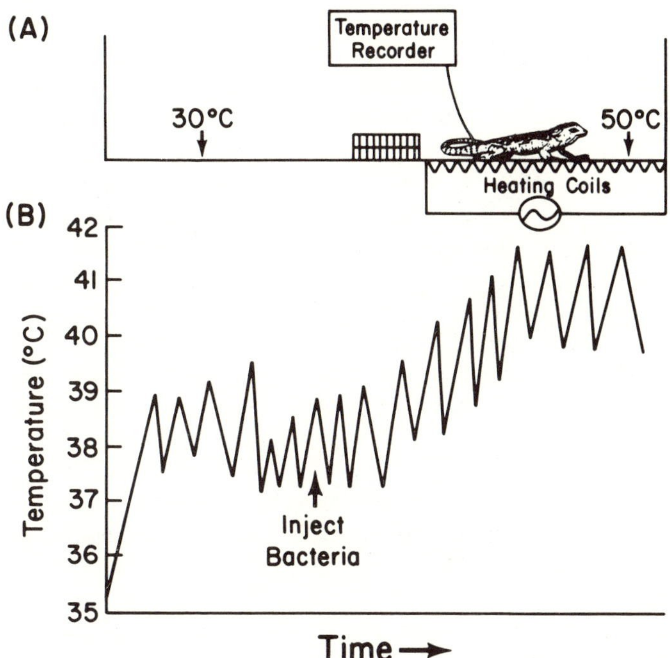

Figure 22. A. Lizard (*Dipsosaurus dorsalis*) in shuttle box. One end is maintained at 30°C and the other end at 50°C. A bridge separates the two sides. A thermocouple is inserted into the cloaca of the lizard and taped to its tail. As a result, the body temperature of these lizards could be recorded continuously.

B. The lizard's body temperature rises to approximately 39°C (time 0). At that point the lizard moves from the warm side of the shuttle box to the cooler end. As a result, its body temperature falls. At a body temperature of approximately 37.5°C it moves from the cool side of the shuttle box to the warm side. These cycles are repeated many times each day. As a result, the lizard maintains an average body temperature of approximately 38°C. Within a few hours following inoculation with pathogenic bacteria, the lizard begins to regulate its body temperature at higher temperatures. For example, now the lizard remains on the warm side of the shuttle box until its body temperature is above 41°C and returns to the warm side when its body temperature falls below 40°C. As a result, the lizard now has an average body temperature of approximately 41°C.

tion (either in the sensory or integrating limbs of the thermoregulatory reflex), then it is possible that pyrogens (fever producing agents) would affect the activity patterns of these neurons. Within the space of one year, three laboratories independently reported that pyrogens do indeed alter the thermosensitivity of these neurons (Wit and Wang 1968; Cabanac et al. 1968; Eisenman 1969). These investigators found that pyrogens decreased the rate of firing of warm-sensitive neurons at essentially all physiological temperatures. Cabanac et al. (1968) also showed that pyrogens caused cold-sensitive neurons to increase their sensitivity to temperature. The antipyretic drug, acetylsalicylate, was shown to return the pyrogen-depressed, warm-sensitive neurons back toward their intitial sensitivity (Wit and Wang 1968) (Figure 23). The results of these studies support the raised set-point theory of fever. At any given temperature, the firing rate of warm-sensitive neurons is depressed and the firing rate of cold-sensitive neurons is elevated by pyrogens. This is what would happen if the organism were hypothermic. As a result, the organism would initiate appropriate responses which would tend to elevate its body temperature.

To summarize, both those experiments involving the physiological and behavioral responses of intact organisms, and those involving electrical recordings of neuronal acitivity, support Liebermeister's claim made over 100 years ago that during fever " 'heat' regulation is adjusted to a higher level." As such, one can differentiate between fever, a regulated rise in body temperature, from other elevations in body temperature, such as those that occur during exposure to a high environmental temperature (hyperthermia). In fever, the organism initiates thermoregulatory responses designed to maintain an elevated body temperature, whereas in hyperthermia, these thermoregulatory responses are all designed to return body temperature to a lower level (see Figure 20).

Biology of Fever

Naturally occurring fevers result from bacterial or viral in-

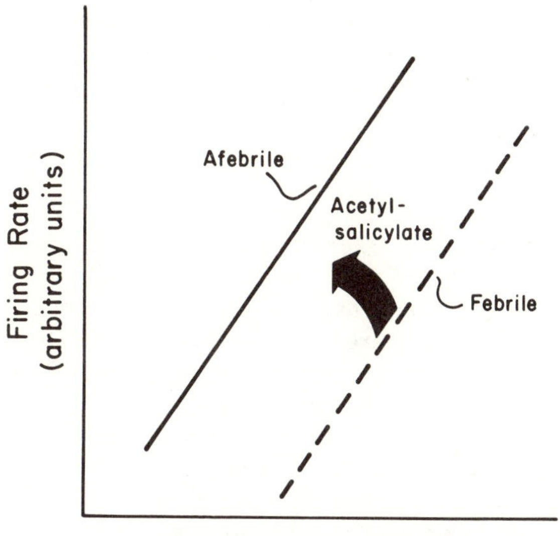

Figure 23. Firing rate vs. temperature of warm-sensitive neurons located in the anterior hypothalamus. At any hypothalamic temperature, the neuron's firing rate is greater when the animal is afebrile compared to when it is febrile. The antipyretic drug acetylsalicylate returns the firing rate of these neurons toward their initial thermal sensitivity. (Based on Wit and Wang [1968] and others.)

fections, or from any other antigen-antibody reaction which causes moderate to severe inflammation (such as occurs during hypersensitivity reactions or injuries). The exact chain of events leading to the elevation in set-point is still unclear. It is currently believed that a variety of antigens serves as "activators" for a series of reactions leading to a fever (Atkins and Bodel 1972). In the process of phagocytizing these "activators" (also called "exogenous pyrogens," by some), the host's leukocytes, or related immunologically active phagocytic cells, produce and release a small molecular weight protein known as "leukocytic" or "endogenous" pyrogens. It is this substance which is thought to trigger several biochemical reactions in the brain of the host organism, resulting in the elevation of its temperature set-point. The various components in the pathways leading from the activators to the development of fever are described below.

A. Activators of Fever

i. Endotoxins

Many substances are known to initiate the febrile pathway. The best known, and most intensively studied, are a component of the cell wall of Gram-negative bacteria known as endotoxin. Nowotny (1969) has described over twenty different effects endotoxins have on the host organism. These include a reduction in the number of circulating white blood cells (leukopenia) followed by the production of new white blood cells (leukocytosis), a protection against irradiation, an enhancement of nonspecific immunological resistance, a reduction in serum iron levels, a lowering of blood pressure, and fever. Endotoxins consist of various components, with a lipopolysaccharide portion considered to be most critical in initiating most of the physiological events attributable to endotoxins. These lipopolysaccharides consist of three regions, two being polysaccharides, and the third being a lipid. Evidence indicates that it is this lipid, called "lipid A," which is responsible for many of the effects of endotoxins (Luderitz et al. 1973). Lipid A has been isolated from endotoxins by two methods. The first involves the use of mutant strains of bacterias which are defective in their synthesis of their cell walls, producing essentially normal lipid A without the associated polysaccharides. The other method involves the use of various biochemical extraction procedures to isolate lipid A.

Phagocytosis of the lipid A component of the cell wall triggers the release of endogenous pyrogens. Endogenous pyrogens will be produced whether the endotoxin comes from dead or live bacteria. The fact that dead Gram-negative bacteria are just as potent as live bacteria in initiating a fever has been known for over 100 years (see the excellent review by Bennett and Beeson 1950).

In 1855, Panum extracted from putrefying solutions endotoxins which when injected into dogs produced several symptoms including fever. In 1866, Frese showed that boiling did not impair the fever-producing capacity of decomposing tissues. Some of the major advances in understanding the relationship between bacteria and fever came as the result of the increasing practice, in the early 1900s, of injecting drugs into patients. Often, when these drugs were given intravenously or subcutaneously, a fever resulted. Hort and Penfold (1911) showed that injections of the solute alone (generally a salt solution) led to all of the characteristics we now know are attributable to endotoxins. It was suggested by some that these fevers were proportional to the volume of the injected salt. Hort and Penfold demonstrated, however, that injections of distilled water, by themselves, also led to a fever. They suggested that it was contamination with bacteria that was responsible for these inflammatory reactions. They also found that autoclaving the saline or water at 120°C failed to eliminate the pyrogenicity. Distilled water, on the other hand, if injected shortly after being collected, was not pyrogenic; but, after being exposed to room air for a short period of time, bacterial growth occurred, and the solution once again became pyrogenic.

Many other investigators worked in this area over the next fifteen years, but it was the careful work of Seibert which demonstrated conclusively that numerous fevers attributable to salts, vaccines, and other injectable agents were in fact due to a heat stable bacterial product, or endotoxin. Seibert (1923) systematically investigated the potential causes of fever, excluding such impurities as inorganic salts, glass dissolved from the container, gases from the air, etc. She argued in favor of the theory that bacterial contaminants were the pyrogenic agents by noting that "non-fever-producing waters may spontaneously become fever-producing after standing at least four days under non-sterile conditions, and bacteria can be isolated from such waters" (Seibert 1925). In a subsequent paper, Bourn and Seibert (1925) were able to isolate from these waters some of these fever-producing bacteria.

Although the effects of bacterial contamination of solutions used in injections (whether or not they have been autoclaved) have been known to be pyrogenic (as well as inducing a host of other reactions attributable to endotoxins) since the early 1900s, it is still surprising to observe how widespread is the misconception that autoclaving destroys endotoxins. As a result, it is still common for experimental biologists to inject their animals with solutions prepared from tap or distilled water which undoubtedly is contaminated with a multitude of bacteria and their by-products. Clearly, injections which contain contaminated water can lead to spurious results.

Until recently, the most sensitive means for determining if a solution was contaminated with endotoxin was to inject the solution into an animal and observe whether a fever developed. The laboratory rabbit was generally used for bioassaying for endotoxin. The use of the laboratory rabbit for pyrogen testing is probably based on the work of Seibert, who, in the process of investigating the causes of fever, made thousands of observations on the febrile response of this animal. She found that the laboratory rabbit was an excellent animal to use to test for pyrogenicity of contaminated solutions. For example, doses as low as 0.0001 μg/kg of endotoxin can induce a fever in these animals (Snell and Atkins 1968). Man, dog, cat, and horse are also about equally sensitive to endotoxins, whereas, for reasons I will go into later, many rodents (rats, mice, etc.) are not particularly sensitive to these substances.

In recent years, the measurement of endotoxins has involved the "*Limulus* assay." *Limulus polyphemus* (the horseshoe crab) is a marine invertebrate distantly related to spiders. In 1956, Bang noted that an injection of Gram-negative bacteria caused fatal intravascular coagulation in *Limulus*. The blood of *Limulus* contains only one type of cell—the amebocyte—and on exposure to endotoxins, these amebocytes produce and liberate a clottable protein (Levin and Bang 1968). The rate of this gelation was found to be proportional to the amount of endotoxin present. Apparently, endotoxins activate an enzyme which in turn initiates clotting or gelation (Young et al. 1972).

Levin and Bang (1968), in discussing the adaptive role of

Limulus' exquisite sensitivity to endotoxin, noted that horseshoe crabs live in an environment which exposes them to numerous Gram-negative pathogenic bacteria. If these bacteria were able to break through their external barriers and penetrate into their vascular system (as could occur following injury), the amebocytes would initiate gelation, thus immobilizing these pathogens. Furthermore, since amebocytes have also been shown to have bactericidal activity (kill bacteria), these "localized" bacteria would then be killed. In these two respects, amebocytes are similar to mammalian platelets.

Based on the ability of *Limulus* blood to clot on contact with endotoxin, Levin and Bang (1964) developed an in vitro assay for endotoxin. The presence of endotoxin was determined by visually observing the degree of gelation after combining an unknown solution with *Limulus* blood. Recently, this test has been made more objective and sensitive so that picogram quantitites of pyrogen can now be detected (Mears et al. 1977).

When a rabbit is injected with endotoxin, or with dead or live Gram-negative bacteria, a fever will develop after a fifteen-to-thirty-minute latency (Beeson 1947a). This latency varies between species, with a latency of about one hour in human beings and as much as three or more hours in birds (Figure 24). With repeated injections of endotoxin, the magnitude and duration of the fever tends to diminish. To compare fevers, Beeson (1947a) calculated a "fever index." He did this by taking as a baseline the animal's core temperature at the time of injection and measuring with a planimeter (integrating) the area enclosed between this baseline and the elevated temperature. The fever index, as used by Beeson, yielded arbitrary units, which were useful in comparing fevers between different animals and between the same animal at different times. As seen in Figure 25, the fever index falls rapidly with repeated injections. Other laboratories have often used the fever index to express the fever, in some units, for a given period of time (Bornstein and Woods 1969; Kaiser and Wood 1962). For example, a fever index 60 is essentially the same as that used by Beeson,

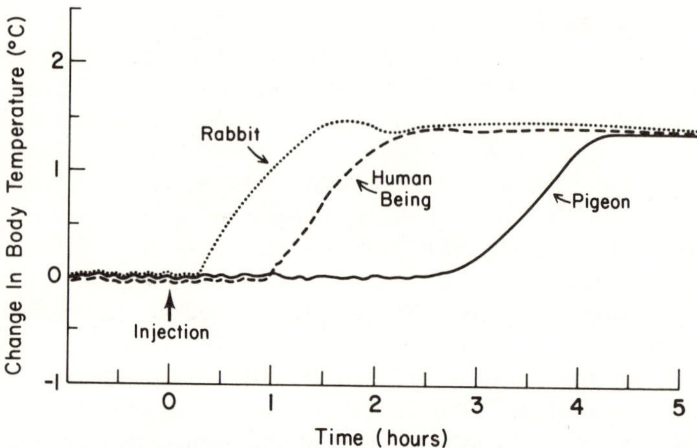

Figure 24. Diagrammatic representation of the latencies associated with injections of endotoxins in rabbits, people, and birds. Note that the rabbit develops a fever within thirty minutes following an injection of endotoxin, whereas this latency can be three hours or more in birds.

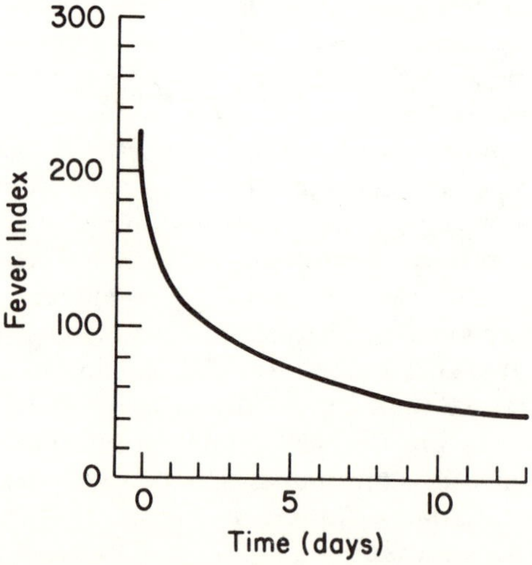

Figure 25. Fever indices of eighty-five rabbits vs. time in days. Each rabbit received a daily injection of purified bacterial pyrogens. Notice that by day 2 the fever index had already begun to fall. (Data redrawn from Beeson 1947a.)

with the exception that the calculations are made for only the initial sixty minutes following the injection. Since a fever index is nothing more than the average fever (for any given time period) multiplied by some constant, one wonders why the magnitude and duration of fever were not simply expressed in terms of average fever in degrees centigrade, rather than in some arbitrary terms. In recent years, the term "fever-index" has been used with decreasing frequency.

The explanations for both the latency period following an injection of endotoxins and the development of tolerance following repeated injections of endotoxins are related to the phagocytosis of the endotoxins and the subsequent production of endogenous pyrogens by various types of effector cells of the immune system. These will be discussed later in this chapter.

An interesting phenomenon occurs in rats following injections with endotoxins. Many investigators have reported that injections with endotoxins resulted not in a fever, but rather in a fall in body temperature in rodents (van Miert and Frens 1968; Winter and Nuss 1963). Others have shown that injections of endotoxins do produce fevers in rats (Avery and Penn 1974; Feldberg and Saxena 1975). No satisfactory explanation has been given for these contradictory results. Recently, a curious phenomenon was reported concerning endotoxin-induced fever in rats (Splawinski et al. 1977). The initial injections of endotoxin did not change the body temperature of the rats, but when the injection was repeated forty-eight hours later, a fever developed. With increasing injections, the magnitude and duration of the fevers diminished, demonstrating tolerance (Figure 26). Splawinski et al. removed blood samples from rats two, five, fifteen, and ninety minutes following injections with endotoxin and tested the pyrogenicity of this blood using the laboratory rabbit as a bioassay. The results of these experiments are seen in Figure 27. When endotoxin was injected for the first time into rats, the fever-inducing activity of rat plasma was greatly diminished with time. When endotoxin was injected for the second time into these rats, the fever-

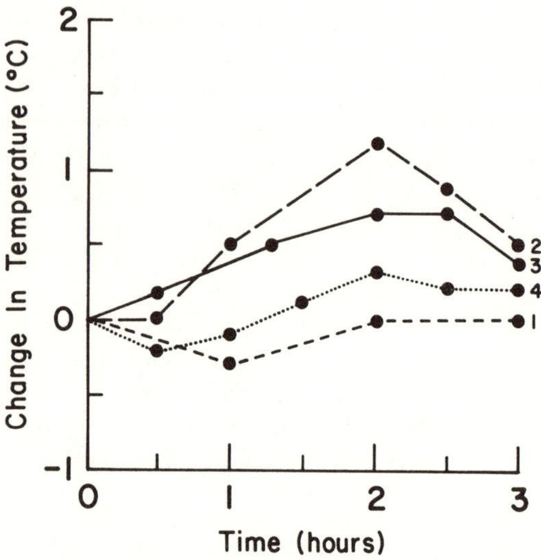

Figure 26. Effect of intravenous injection of endotoxin on the core temperature of rats. The first injection of endotoxin (1) produced no change in body temperature. A fever developed following the second and third (2 and 3) injections of endotoxin, but no fever developed following the fourth injection of endotoxin (4). (Data redrawn from Splawinski et al. 1977.)

inducing activity of the rat plasma was unchanged with time. On the assumption that the fever-inducing activity of rat plasma is due to the circulating endotoxin, they concluded that the absence of fever following the initial injection of endotoxin might be related to the rapid loss or detoxification of endotoxin. The absence of this detoxifying activity following the second injection (at forty-eight hours), they suggested, is related to the inactivation of this detoxification process. The question of why different laboratories have found such divergent results (either a rise, a fall, or no change in body temperature) following injections of endotoxin into rats has yet to be resolved, but might be related to the above phenomenon.

ii. Gram-positive Bacteria

Although Gram-positive bacteria are not thought to possess

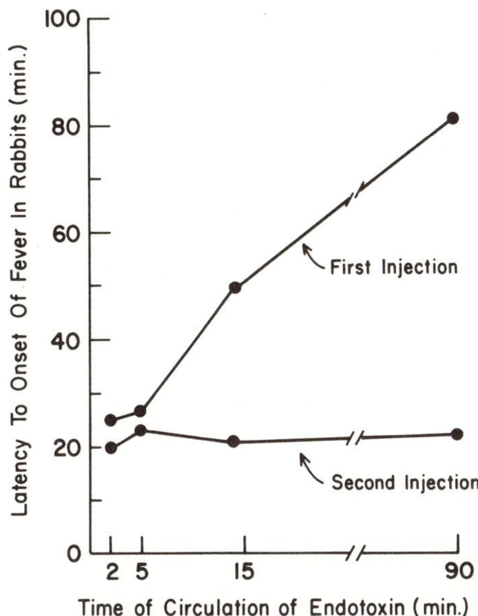

Figure 27. Latency to onset of fever in rabbits (following injection with plasma removed from rats) vs. the time of circulation of endotoxin in rats. Each rat was injected with endotoxin and after two, five, fifteen, and ninety minutes, a sample of each rat's plasma was injected into rabbits. Notice that after an initial injection of endotoxin into these rats (First Injection), the pyrogenicity of their plasma diminished rapidly. For example, within fifteen minutes, a sample of their plasma produced a fever in rabbits after a latency of fifty minutes. Following a second injection (Second Injection) of endotoxin into these rats, their plasma remained pyrogenic for at least ninety minutes. Notice that injections of this plasma into rabbits produced fevers within twenty-five minutes whether the plasma was removed at two minutes or at ninety minutes following injection with endotoxin. (Redrawn from Splawinski et al. 1977.)

endotoxins, these bacteria are still pyrogenic (Snell and Atkins 1968). Atkins and Freedman (1963) have shown that a variety of Gram-positive organisms, including *Staphylococcus sp*. and *Pneumococcus sp*., are pyrogenic in the laboratory rabbit. As in the case of Gram-negative bacteria, heat-killed gram-positive bacteria will also cause fevers.

The onset of fever following an injection of Gram-positive

bacteria is considerably longer compared to that of an intravenous injection of endotoxin or Gram-negative bacteria. Hort and Penfold (1912) reported that fever developed several hours after inoculation with Gram-positive bacteria. Atkins and Freedman (1963) have shown that intravenous injections of live or dead Gram-positive bacteria will induce a fever within forty-five to sixty minutes (Figure 28). Another difference between Gram-negative and Gram-positive fevers is that daily injections of Gram-positive cocci or bacilli failed to diminish the febrile response in rabbits, suggesting that tolerance to Gram-positive bacteria does not occur (Atkins and Freedman 1963). As in endotoxin fevers, Gram-positive fevers are also thought to be mediated via the production of endogenous pyrogens.

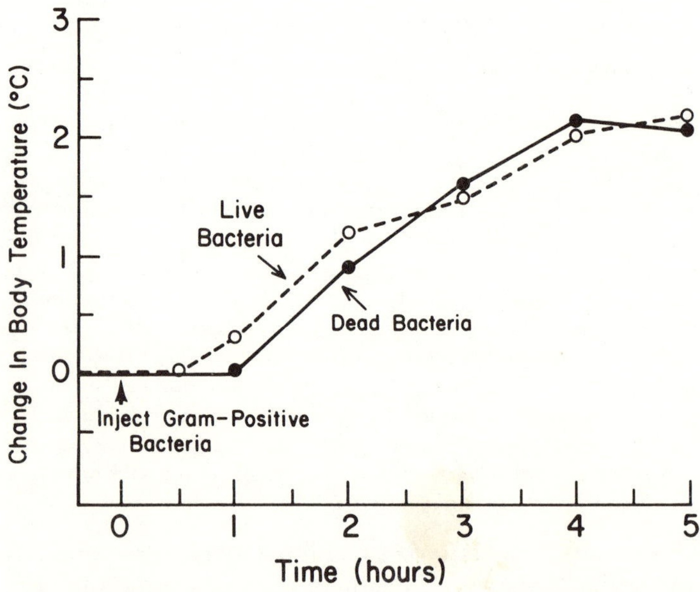

Figure 28. Effects of injection of dead or live Gram-positive bacteria (*Staphylococcus aureus*) on the body temperature of rabbits. Note that after forty-five minutes to one hour, a fever develops in response to an intravenous infusion of either dead of live bacteria. (Based on Atkins and Freedman 1963.)

iii. Viruses

Because of the difficulties involved in working with viruses, there have been few studies concerning virus-induced fever. In 1949, Wagner et al. showed that intravenous injections of three types of viruses (two strains of influenza and one strain of Newcastle disease virus) led to fevers in rabbits. These fevers began within one to two hours and continued for as long as twenty-four hours. Heating these viruses to temperatures as low as 60° or 70°C destroyed their pyrogenicity. Whereas injections with bacteria result in a decrease in the circulating white blood cells known as granulocytes, injections with viruses result in a decrease in another type of white blood cell, the lymphocyte (Wagner et al. 1949).

Tolerance to viruses occurs rapidly. An intravenous injection of viruses twenty-four hours after the initial injection failed to produce a fever in laboratory rabbits (Bennett et al. 1949). Viruses heated to temperatures below 60°C conferred tolerance as readily as did unheated preparations. In 1953, Wagner reported that mumps virus also induced fevers in rabbits, and that tolerance also occurred within twenty-four hours of the initial injection. An interesting finding in this study was that he found cross-tolerance to viral pyrogens. That is, when mumps virus was injected on day 1, injection with influenza virus on day 2 failed to produce a fever, and vice versa.

Viruses are also thought to induce a fever via the production of endogenous pyrogens (Atkins and Huang 1958; King 1964). After injecting viruses into rabbits, an endogenous pyrogenlike substance was found circulating in the sera of these febrile rabbits. Injections of this sera produced fevers in recipient rabbits. Atkins et al. (1964) have shown that in vitro incubations of rabbit blood cells with purified parainfluenza virus led to the production of endogenous pyrogens, which were indistinguishable from bacterially induced endogenous pyrogens.

iv. Hypersensitivity Reactions

Although antigens are difficult to define, in general terms they are thought of as any substance which induces the production of antibodies. Antibodies, in turn, are specialized proteins which are synthesized in response to contact of specialized white blood cells (lymphocytes) with these antigens. One type of lymphocyte secretes antibodies (gamma globulins or immunoglobulins), which are released into the blood or other body fluids, and forms the basis for what is known as "humoral" immunity. Another type of lymphocyte has antibodylike molecules on its surface ("cell-bound antibody") and is responsible for "cell mediated" immunity (Roitt 1974).

The combination of specific antibodies with specific antigens (in humoral immunity), or of "sensitized" lymphocytes with specific antigens (in cell mediated immunity), triggers a series of reactions which can result in (1) an enhancement of the inflammatory response resulting in phagocytosis of the antigens, (2) direct killing of microorganisms without prior phagocytosis, and (3) neutralization of bacterial toxins and viruses (Vander et al. 1975).

Following initial contact with an antigen, the organism slowly produces antibodies or sensitized lymphocytes specific for that antigen. The individual is said to be immunologically primed or sensitized (Roitt 1974). In humoral immunity, on second exposure to these antigens, antibodies are rapidly produced. In cell mediated immunity, lymphocytes are probably already sensitized. In any event, these antibodies or sensitized lymphocytes trigger the events listed above. Occasionally, this response to antigen is heightened to an extent that is harmful to the well-being of the host (Barrett 1974). This is known as hypersensitivity. Hypersensitivity reactions can lead to edema, swelling, tissue necrosis, or death, as well as many other side effects, including fever.

Hypersensitivity reactions are thought to be responsible for many fevers seen clinically. For example, hypersensitivity resulting in fever often occurs in sensitized subjects in response to infectious agents such as bacteria, viruses, protozoans, and fungi, or to such noninfectious agents as drugs, toxins present in some ingested food, transplanted tissues, etc. (Snell 1971).

There are apparently two separate pathways for the development of hypersensitivity-induced fevers (see reviews by Snell 1971 or Bodel 1974). The first involves the reaction of antigens with circulating antibodies in the previously sensitized organism. For example, Farr et al. (1954a) have shown that rabbits which are sensitized to bovine serum albumen (BSA) would respond to repeated injections of BSA by developing a fever. This response was qualitatively similar to that seen following injections of endotoxins, raising the question of whether endotoxin-induced fevers might actually be attributable to a hypersensitivity reaction. Snell (1971) compared endotoxin-induced fevers with hypersensitivity-induced fevers and noted that although there are many similarities, there are also some important differences between the two. He concluded that despite a superficial resemblance, an endotoxin-induced fever is unlikely to be a hypersensitivity fever. The other pathway for hypersensitivity-induced fevers involves what is known as delayed hypersensitivity and is caused by cell mediated, rather than humoral, processes.

Both types of hypersensitivity-induced fevers are thought to initiate the fever via the production of endogenous pyrogens. Hall and Atkins (1959) and Jahanovsky (1959) found that rabbits which were made febrile by a hypersensitivity reaction to tuberculin had circulating endogenous pyrogenlike substances which were indistinguishable in their biological effects from endogenous pyrogens obtained by injections of endotoxins. Hypersensitivity reactions in rabbits to human serum albumin also led to circulating endogenous pyrogenlike substances (Root and Wolff 1968).The exact mechanism by which hypersensitivity reactions lead to the production of endogenous pyrogens is unknown, although in delayed hypersensitivity it has been speculated that the combination of antigens with "cell-bound antibody" causes these lymphocytes to produce a nonpyrogenic intermediate called "lymphokine" (Bodel 1974; Atkins and Francis 1977). It is speculated that this "lymphokine" induces the production of endogenous pyrogens from special types of effector cells, resulting in a fever.

v. Tumors

Fever is associated with many types of malignancies. Although these fevers are sometimes attributed to secondary bacterial or viral infections, they often occur without any identifiable infectious agent. Several hypotheses have been proposed to explain tumor-induced fevers (see review by Bodel 1974). Some of these are (1) the production of some toxin from the tumor, (2) tissue necrosis with the release of some pyrogenic materials, and (3) an undiagnosed infection.

Bodel (1974) has shown that pyrogens are produced during an in vitro incubation of various types of tumor cells with serum obtained from the same host. Her studies demonstrated that this pyrogen substance was probably an endogenous pyrogen. The specific activator for tumor-induced fever is still unknown. Bodel suggests that the activator might be a virus, or some other carcinogenic agent, or more like a hypersensitivity response of the host to some component of the tumor.

B. Endogenous Pyrogens

i. Introduction

As evident from the preceding section, all activators of fever (endotoxins from Gram-negative bacteria, Gram-positive bacteria, viruses, hypersensitivity reactions to various antigens, and tumors) appear to induce the formation of endogenous pyrogens from the host's own cells. The first clear demonstrations that endogenous pyrogens were substances distinct from endotoxin, or some other activator of fever, were made by Beeson (1948), and Bennett and Beeson (1953a, b). Beeson (1948) reported that when a sterile, pyrogen-free physiologic salt solution was injected into the peritoneal cavity of rabbits, several types of cells migrated into this fluid. When this peritoneal exudate was removed, four types of cells was found—erythrocytes, lymphocytes, macrophages, and polymorphonuclear granulocytes. These latter three cell types are often collectively known as white blood cells. The granulocytes, when subjected to mechanical disruption or lysis, liberated a substance into the solution which, when injected into rabbits, produced a fever. The erythrocytes, lymphocytes, and macrophages failed to produce a pyrogenic substance. Beeson found that the pyrogenic material released from the granulocytes was rendered ineffective when heated to temperatures which denatured proteins. Bennett and Beeson (1953a, b) investigated this pyrogenic substance in more detail. Whereas their studies indicated that endogenous pyrogens were produced only by granulocytes, they believed that other immunologically active cells were probably also involved in the production of these endogenous pyrogens. They noted that Bennett and Cluff (1952) had treated rabbits with nitrogen mustard, an agent which suppresses the formation of polymorphonuclear granulocytes. These animals still responded to bacterial pyrogens and other activators of fever by developing a fever. Later studies by Herion et al. (1961) resulted in somewhat opposite results. They found that rabbits which were made severely leukopenic, to the extent that they had no circulating granulocytes (other than basophilic granulocytes), failed to develop a fever in response to injection with endotoxin. Herion and his associates found a positive correlation between the numbers of circulating granulocytes (other than the basophils) and the magnitude of the febrile response to endotoxins. These leukopenic rabbits still responded to injections of endogneous pyrogens (from donor rabbits) by developing a fever. Despite these data, there is considerable evidence which supports Bennett's and Beeson's belief that many other types of cells are also capable of producing endogenous pyrogens. These data will be discussed later.

ii. Comparison between Endogenous Pyrogens and Endotoxin

Endogenous pyrogens are low molecular weight (15-40,000) proteins. Since they are proteins, they are readily denatured or inactivated by high temperatures. Although endogenous pyrogens are sometimes confused with endotoxins, a comparison of these substances (Table 2) serves to highlight the many differences between the two.

As seen from Table 2, an endogenous pyrogen (a protein)

Table 2. Comparison of An Endogenous Pyrogen with Endotoxin

Property	*Endogenous Pyrogen*	*Endotoxin*
Heat Stability	Labile (generally inactivated by temperatures as low as 56°C)	Stabile
Chemical Composition	Protein	Lipopolysaccharide
Latency	Short	Long
Tolerance	Little or no tolerance to repeated injections	Tolerance develops to repeated injections

is much more sensitive to heat than is an endotoxin (a lipopolysaccharide). Often, if one is concerned whether a preparation of an endogenous pyrogen is contaminated with bacterial products such as endotoxins, the preparation is heated (perhaps at 80° or 90°C) for thirty minutes. If injection of the preparation no longer induces a fever in the test animal, then one can safely conclude that it was not contaminated with endotoxin.

Another property of endogenous pyrogens is that the latency from the time of injection to the initiation of the fever is considerably shorter than in endotoxin-induced fevers. It is not uncommon for an intravenous injection of an endogenous pyrogen into a rabbit to produce a fever in less than ten minutes, whereas this latency can be twenty to thirty minutes following an intravenous injection of endotoxin. The explanation for the shorter latency with endogenous pyrogens is, of course, that endotoxins must first stimulate the production and release of endogenous pyrogens before the fever can develop. Therefore, when an endogenous pyrogen is injected, the first step has been removed along the pathway toward the development of fever.

An animal develops little tolerance to endogenous pyrogens, whereas, as discussed briefly above, repeated injections of endotoxin result in tolerance. The question of why tolerance develops to endotoxin is an interesting one and is related in part to the enhanced clearance, or removal, of endotoxin from the blood with repeated injections. An organism which becomes tolerant to the fever-inducing properties of endotoxins will also become refractory to many of the other effects of endotoxins (shock, lethality, etc.). Beeson (1947b) found that the reticulo-endothelial system is extremely important in removing endotoxin from the blood. The reticulo-endothelial system is a general term for the various types of cells which have the common function of being phagocytic. These cells, which line many of the vascular and lymphatic passages, are found in such tissues as bone marrow, spleen, liver, and lymph nodes.

Certain colloidal agents such as thorium dioxide (Thorotrast) are thought to block the reticulo-endothelial system. Beeson (1947b) found that in rabbits, whose febrile responses to endotoxins were markedly reduced as the result of repeated injections, injections of thorium dioxide led to an enhancement of the febrile response. Furthermore, he reported that pyrogenic substances disappeared from the blood more rapidly in tolerant rabbits than in control rabbits. When thorium dioxide was injected into tolerant rabbits, the speed of disappearance of pyrogens from the blood was reduced. Beeson (1947a) also reported that rabbits which had become unresponsive to endotoxin from one species of bacteria were found to be somewhat tolerant to endotoxins from other species of bacteria and that tolerance was not correlated with specific antibody titers, confirming an earlier study by Favorite and Morgan (1942).

These important studies of Beeson have been largely confirmed. For example, Atkins and Wood (1955) have studied the rate of clearance of Gram-negative bacteria in unsensitized (those which had received no injections of bacteria), sensitized (those which had received one or two injections of bacteria), and tolerant (those that had received daily injections of bacteria for seven or eight days) rabbits. After injections of bacteria, blood was removed from these rabbits and serum was injected into recipient rabbits. They found that rabbits which received serum from unsensitized rabbits developed greater fevers than did those rabbits which received serum from sensitized rabbits, and that rabbits receiving serum from tolerant donors did not develop a fever.

Several other laboratories, however, suggested that humoral factors (antibodies) might still play a role in tolerance to endotoxins. For example, Farr et al. (1954b) demonstrated that partial tolerance could be passively transferred from tolerant animals to unsensitized animals by injecting serum from tolerant donors. Benacerraf et al. (1959), using radioactively labeled bacteria, confirmed Beeson's findings that the removal of these bacteria from the blood was related to the phagocytic activity of the reticulo-endothelial system, particularly in the liver and spleen; but he also found that the rate of clearance of these bacteria by the reticulo-endothelial system was related to the level of serum antibodies. Jenkin and Rowley (1961) demonstrated that serum factors are important and presented evidence that opsonins play a role in endotoxin clearance. (Opsonins are antibodies which attach themselves to an antigen and result in an enhancement of phagocytosis.) These results have been confirmed by studies from several other laboratories (see reviews by Snell 1971 and Atkins and Bodel 1974).

As a result of these findings, Greisman et al. (1963) suggested a dual system for tolerance to pyrogenic substances. One is related to the clearance of bacteria by the reticulo-endothelial system, occurs fairly rapidly, and is unrelated to the production of antibodies. The other is related to the production of opsonins which facilitate phagocytosis (also in the reticulo-endothelial system). Wolff et al. (1965) reported data which support this hypothesis. They found that the suppression of serum antibodies (using drugs) still led to the development of tolerance and therefore concluded that serum antibodies could not be the sole factor responsible for tolerance. These data supported earlier observations that patients with agammaglobulinemia (antibody deficiency) could still be made tolerant to endotoxins (Figure 29) (Good and Varco 1955).

In 1968, Dinarello et al. reported that specialized phagocytic cells found in the liver (Kupffer cells) produced an endogenous pyrogen when incubated with bacteria or endotoxin. They suggested that a third component of tolerance is related to the production of an endogenous pyrogen by these Kupffer cells. When Kupffer cells from endotoxin tolerant rabbits were incubated with endotoxin, less endogen-

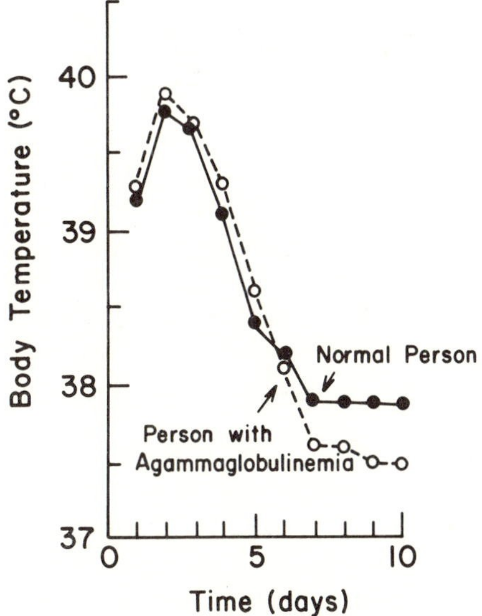

Figure 29. Development of tolerance in a normal person and in one with agammaglobulinemia. Each person was inoculated each day with endotoxin and his body temperatures were recorded. The person with the antibody deficiency failed to develop serum antibodies to the endotoxin, whereas the normal person developed high titers to the endotoxin. In both individuals, tolerance to the intravenous injection of endotoxin developed, indicating that tolerance (diminished febrile response to repeated injections) is not dependent on antibody production. (Data redrawn from Good and Varco 1955.)

ous pyrogen was produced. Furthermore, incubation of Kupffer cells from unsensitized rabbits with endotoxin and serum from tolerant animals also led to a reduction in the amount of endogenous pyrogens produced, suggesting a humoral component to this reduction in pyrogens by the Kupffer cells. Greisman and Woodward (1970) confirmed these findings and found that part of the endogenous pyrogens produced in endotoxin-induced fevers comes from extrahepatic sources (mostly granulocytes) and part from hepatic sources (Kupffer cells).

Our current understanding of the process of tolerance to endotoxin-induced fevers can therefore be summarized as follows:

1. Tolerance results in the increased rate of removal of endotoxin by the reticulo-endothelial system. There are apparently two mechanisms behind this increased clearance. One is related to some change in the reticulo-endothelial system and is thought to occur independently of serum antibodies. The other is related to serum antibodies known as opsonins. These cause the circulating endotoxins to be more easily phagocytized by cells of the reticulo-endothelial system.

2. Tolerance also results in Kupffer cells producing less endogenous pyrogen. This decrease in the production of endogenous pyrogens can be induced by humoral factors. It is unknown whether some component of this refractoriness is also related to some nonhumoral factor.

Tolerance also occurs in response to repeated injections of other activators of fever (e.g. antigens leading to hypersensitivity reactions, viruses, etc.). The mechanisms behind tolerance to these agents have been less well studied than tolerance to endotoxins. Briefly, tolerance to hypersensitivity-induced fevers appears to be related to changes in the interactions between antigens and antibodies by a process called desensitization. Tolerance to viruses is thought to be related to a decreased production of endogenous pyrogens. For more details on the mechanisms of tolerance to the activators of fever, the reader is referred to the excellent reviews by Snell (1971) and Atkins and Bodel (1974).

Tolerance, to some extent, also occurs to repeated injections of endogenous pyrogens (Bornstein et al. 1963). It is thought that an injection of endogenous pyrogens induces a fever by two pathways. One is by the direct effect of the endogenous pyrogens on the thermoregulatory centers in the brain (leading to a rise in the set-point); the other is by a stimulation of immunologically active cells to produce increased endogenous pyrogens. Apparently, with repeated injections of endogenous pyrogens, this internal production of endogenous pyrogens becomes diminished (Bornstein et al. 1963). It is unknown what mechanism is responsible for the decreased production of endogenous pyrogens by the host, although this might be related to mechanisms behind the tolerance to other activators such as desensitization.

iii. Cell Sources and Mechanism of Production of Endogenous Pyrogens

Although the data of Herion and his associates (1961) pointed toward the conclusion that circulating polymorphonuclear granulocytes were the only producers of endogenous pyrogens, much data have accumulated indicating that many other types of immunologically active cells are also capable of producing endogenous pyrogens. For example, besides the granulocytes, cells such as monocytes, macrophages, and Kupffer cells have all been shown to produce endogenous pyrogens when incubated in vitro with various types of activating agents (Atkins and Bodel 1974).

Endogenous pyrogens can be produced in vitro by several methods. One involves obtaining white blood cells from the peritoneal cavity. About 200 milliliters (or more) of sterile pyrogen-free saline is injected into the abdomen of an animal weighing between 2 and 3 kg. After a few hours, this fluid is removed and is generally found to contain a large number of polymorphonuclear granulocytes (Mudd et al. 1929; Ponder and MacLeod 1938). Apparently these exudate leukocytes have already been activated, since incubation of these cells in saline (at about 37°C for several hours) results in the release of an endogenous pyrogen into the medium (see, for example, Bornstein and Woods 1969). Often an additional stimulant, such as shellfish glycogen, is added to the saline infusate (Kozak et al. 1968). The addition of this substance is thought to serve as a second activator (the first being the presence of saline in the peritoneum) and tends to increase the yield of this endogenous pyrogen. The "peritoneal exudate" method of obtaining white blood cells has been widely used in investigations involving the production of endogenous pyrogens. Leukocytes from rabbits, cats, dogs, goats, and lizards obtained from peritoneal exudates have all been shown to produce and release endogenous pyrogens (Bornstein and Woods 1969; Bernheim and Kluger 1977).

Endogenous pyrogens have also been produced in vitro by white blood cells obtained directly from the blood. These leukocytes, unlike those obtained from peritoneal exudates, are not activated. As a result, incubation of these cells in saline will not yield an appreciable amount of endogenous pyrogens. The addition of some activating agent to the incubating medium (such as Gram-negative or Gram-positive bacteria) results in the production and release of endogenous pyrogens (Bodel et al. 1973). White blood cells obtained by this method from rabbits and human beings have been shown to produce endogenous pyrogens (Bodel and Atkins 1966). Using similar methods, other cells (such as Kupffer cells and monocytes), when activated, will also produce endogenous pyrogens.

The endogenous pyrogens produced by different cell types are not identical. Dinarello et al. (1974) have shown that incubation of activated human blood monocytes resulted in an endogenous pyrogen which was different from the endogenous pyrogen obtained from activated human blood granulocytes. Monocyte-endogenous pyrogen was about twice the size and about forty times as pyrogenic as granulocyte-endogenous pyrogen. The patterns of fever produced by these two types of endogenous pyrogens were also different.

Endogenous pyrogens from the same cell type, but from different species, are not identical. Dinarello et al. (1974) also compared the characteristics of human granulocyte endogenous pyrogens with that of rabbit granulocyte endogenous pyrogens and found that while they were similar, there were distinct differences—the human endogenous pyrogens were larger, more acidic, and more alkaline resistant.

It is interesting to note that even though endogenous pyrogens might have slightly different species-specific characteristics, endogenous pyrogens from one species will, when injected into another species, induce a fever. For example, endogenous pyrogens derived from dogs and cats produced a fever in rabbits; endogenous pyrogens from dogs and rabbits produced a fever in cats; endogenous pyrogens from a dog produced a fever in a goat and a sheep (Bornstein and Woods 1969). These data demonstrated that endogenous pyrogens are cross-species reactive. Bornstein and Woods did find, however, that the febrile response to these "heterologous" endogenous pyrogens was markedly diminished compared to the response produced by equal doses of "homologous" endogenous pyrogens (endogenous pyrogens derived from, and injected into, the same species). More recently, Bernheim and Kluger (1977) have shown that endogenous pyrogens from rabbit exudate leukocytes will produce a fever when injected into lizards, thus demonstrating cross-class reactivity.

Much of what is known about the actual production and release of endogenous pyrogens is based on studies involving activated polymorphonuclear granulocytes. Granulocytes which are disrupted prior to activation generally produce a small quantity of endogenous pyrogens (Atkins and Bodel 1974). The release of this endogenous pyrogen, from activated cells, takes place over a period of several hours and is temperature dependent. These findings suggest that the endogenous pyrogen might be synthesized after the leukocytes are stimulated by some activating agent. In 1970, papers appeared from three independent laboratories which showed that production of endogenous pyrogens was dependent on protein synthesis. Inhibitors of protein synthesis, such as puromycin, cycloheximide, and actinomycin-D, were all found to prevent the synthesis of endogenous pyrogens in blood leukocytes (Moore et al. 1970; Nordlund and Root 1970; Bodel 1970). Hahn et al. (1970), however, found that puromycin did not block the production of endogenous pyrogens from exudate leukocytes. Apparently, since these leukocytes were already activated, in vivo, they probably had started to produce, but not yet release, the endogenous pyrogen. Moore et al. (1973) have found that after activation the leukocytes can be shown to incorporate radioactively labeled amino acids into the endogenous pyrogen. Apparently, the endogenous pyrogen is still in the form of an inactive precursor even after this initial stage of protein synthesis. Disrupting the leukocytes at this time results in the release of only a small amount of the endogenous pyrogen. The conversion of the inactive precursor to the active form of endogenous pyrogen seems to occur without any further protein synthesis. The mechanism behind the release of the active endogenous pyrogen into the surrounding media is unknown.

Thus, activation of leukocytes triggers the production of an endogenous pyrogen precursor. After this initial phase of protein synthesis, the endogenous pyrogen precursor is converted to the active form of endogenous pyrogen and is secreted by these leukocytes. For more details concerning the mechanism of production of endogenous pyrogens, see Atkins and Bodel (1974).

C. Fever and the Central Nervous System

i. Introduction

There is considerable evidence that the central nervous system is involved in the development of fever. While this might sound like a trivial statement, there is often some confusion about the nature of fever. For example, the definition of fever given in a well-known medical dictionary is that fever is "a bodily temperature above the normal of 37°C" (Stedman 1972). This definition does not allow one to distinguish between the potential peripheral and central effects of pyrogens. As discussed above, there is convincing evidence that a fever involves the raising of the central nervous system's set-point for the regulation of body temperatures. As such, fever (the result of pyrogens affecting the central nervous system) can be distinguished from hyperthermia (the result of excess heat).

ii. Pyrogens and the Brain

Direct evidence that the brain is involved in the development of fever was first shown by King and Wood (1958). These investigators rationalized that if the brain were involved in fever, then an injection of an endogenous pyrogen into the carotid arteries (which lead directly to the ventral surface of the brain) should produce a fever of shorter latency and greater magnitude than one following an injection of endogenous pyrogens into a vein. If pyrogens cause fevers by affecting tissues peripheral to the brain, then there should either be little difference in the fevers between the two routes of injection, or alternately, the intravenous route should actually lead to fevers of shorter latency and greater magnitude. King and Wood found that the injection of an endogenous pyrogen into the carotid arteries of rabbits did produce fevers of shorter latency and greater magnitude than those resulting from injections into veins, confirming that the brain was involved in the development of fever. Furthermore, they also observed that there were no differences in the latencies or magnitudes of the febrile response elicited by the intracarotid and intravenous routes of administration of endotoxin, thus further supporting the belief that endotoxin produces fever by inducing the formation of endogenous pyrogens.

Adler and Joy (1965) later showed that when an endogenous pyrogen was injected directly into the brain (via injection into the cerebrospinal fluid found in the ventricular systems of the brain), the fevers produced were of greater magnitude and duration than those that followed injection of the endogenous pyrogen intravenously. These observations have since been confirmed by several other laboratories. These data, however, did not help to locate with any precision the area(s?) within the brain which are actually affected by these pyrogens. Furthermore, these data still did not exclude the possibility that areas outside the brain are also involved in febrogenesis in response to pyrogens.

Evidence that endogenous pyrogens act directly on sites within the brain, with little effect on sites outside the brain, was provided by Cooper et al. (1967) and by Jackson (1967). Cooper et al. injected small quantities of an endogenous pyrogen into different areas of the brain of rabbits. Only those injections in the preoptic area and anterior hypothalamus (often abbreviated POAH) caused a fever to develop (often within five minutes). The dose of the endogenous pyrogen which caused a fever was less than one-hundredth of that required to produce a fever by intravenous injection. Injections of endotoxin into the POAH also produced a fever; however, the latency averaged about twenty-five minutes. Four of the rabbits which received the injections of endotoxins were killed within twenty to thirty minutes, and many polymorphonuclear leukocytes were found in the region of the injection. Apparently, these leukocytes were phagocytizing the endotoxins and were producing endogenous pyrogen(s?) within these central nervous areas. Jackson (1967), working with cats, reported similar results. These results are compatible with the neurophysiological data (described briefly above) which showed that the activity of thermally sensitive neurons in the POAH was altered by pyrogens.

These data suggest that endogenous pyrogens enter the brain and trigger a fever by some interaction occurring in the POAH. This raises the question of whether endogenous pyrogens can cross the blood brain barrier, and if so, how? The answer to the first question is an equivocal yes. In 1965, Allen published a paper which suggested that an endogenous pyrogen injected into the intracarotid arteries did enter the brain and could be found in the general region of the hypothalamus. In this study, an endogenous pyrogen was produced in a medium containing radioactively labeled iodine. Injection of radioactively labeled serum from control animals led to no detectable traces of radioactivity within the brain. Within sixty minutes following an injection of serum containing this endogenous pyrogen produced in a medium containing radioactive iodine, an area in the posterior hypothalamus (not POAH) could be seen to be radioactive (using radioautographs). However, it was not known whether the radioactivity could be attributed specifically to this endogenous pyrogen.

Recently, more refined techniques have been developed for accurately measuring minute amounts of endogenous pyrogens: a radioimmunoassay (Dinarello et al. 1977). Radioimmunoassays involve the binding of a radioactively labeled antigen to an antibody and are now commonly used to measure the concentrations of many hormones and other substances which heretofore were difficult to quantify. Using the radioimmunoassay for endogenous pyrogens, Dinarello and his colleagues should now be able to determine precisely where these proteins leave the circulation (if at all) and enter the central nervous system. It is possible that under normal physiological conditions, endogenous pyrogens exert their effects on the central nervous system via some intermediate messenger, and as such do not actually enter the brain.

Assuming that the radioautographs in Allen's study were actually recording the presence of an endogenous pyrogen in the posterior hypothalamus, how did the endogenous pyrogen get into this region? Endogenous pyrogens could enter the brain via one of two routes: (1) by being secreted into the cerebrospinal fluid and being carried by bulk flow or by diffusion to the hypothalamus; or (2) by entering the hypothalamus directly from the blood stream. Feldberg et al. (1971) reported that the likely route of entrance of the endogenous pyrogen was via the second route. They perfused the cerebral ventricles of unanesthetized rabbits, from the lateral ventricles to the cisterna magna, with artificial cerebrospinal fluid. The flow rate they chose would effectively remove most of the endogenous pyrogen which might be secreted directly into the cerebrospinal fluid. Following an intravenous injection of an endogenous pyrogen, the fevers which developed in these animals were not different from nonperfused controls in terms of latency, magnitude, or duration. This hypothesis was further supported by studies which indicated that even when the ventricular system was filled with an inert oil (thus essentially preventing any potential exchanges between the cerebrospinal fluid and the hypothalamus), these rabbits still developed fevers of similar latencies to control animals (Cooper and Veale 1972).

In 1971, Rosendorff and Mooney reported that the brainstem of the rabbit is also sensitive to an endogenous pyrogen. They injected minute amounts of an endogenous pyrogen into various regions of the brain and found that the greatest fevers were produced following microinjections into the POAH. The brainstem was somewhat less sensitive to this endogenous pyrogen than the POAH. Injections of this endogenous pyrogen into the posterior hypothalamus caused no fever.

These data concerning endogenous pyrogens and the central nervous system are therefore somewhat paradoxical. Apparently, an endogenous pyrogen is necessary for a fever to develop, and injections of minute amounts of this protein into the POAH or brainstem lead to a fever. The doses necessary to produce a fever via microinjections into these central nervous sites are often less than 1/100 of those necessary to produce a fever by intravenous injections. However, the only study concerning the location of an endogenous pyrogen in the brain, following an intravenous injection, indicated that the endogenous pyrogen migrated, or was transported, to the insensitive posterior hypothalamus and not to the POAH or brainstem. A further complication of these data is provided by the results of lesion studies.

Many investigators have reported that lesioning (or surgically ablating) the POAH has little effect on the febrile response. For example, Veale and Cooper (1975) have reported that following removal of the entire POAH of rabbits, an intravenous injection of an endogenous pyrogen still produced a fever of similar magnitude to that found in control rabbits. Similar results were reported by Andersson et al. (1965) in POAH-lesioned goats. Lipton and Trzcinka (1976) reported that POAH-lesioned monkeys also responded to intravenous injections of pyrogens with fevers indistinguishable from those in control monkeys. Injections of pyrogens into the ventricular system of the brain of these POAH-lesioned monkeys also produced fevers which were indistinguishable from those in control monkeys. Lipton and Trzcinka reviewed much of the literature relating to the febrile responses of POAH-lesioned animals and concluded that the control of fever is not localized solely in the POAH.

An apparent solution to part of this paradox was provided by Rosendorff's and Mooney's results showing that the injections of an endogenous pyrogen into the brainstem could lead to a fever in rabbits. It is, nevertheless, unclear as to how the removal of the POAH (an area of the brain which is thermally sensitive, responsive to pyrogens, and implicated in the integration of thermal information) can result in such a minimal deficit in the febrile response.

iii. Prostaglandins and Fever

Regardless of the exact location of the central nervous sites responsible for the development of a fever, it is still believed that endogenous pyrogens trigger this elevation in set-point. How endogenous pyrogens do this is unclear, although recently a group of lipid acids, prostaglandins, have been implicated in febrogenesis (see Figure 15).

In 1971, Milton and Wendlandt reported that the injection of minute amounts of prostaglandins E_1 and E_2 into the cerebral ventricular system of cats and rabbits produced a fever within a few minutes. Related prostaglandins ($F_2\alpha$, A_1, etc.) failed to produce a fever. Hales et al. (1973) and Feldberg and Saxena (1975) showed that intraventricular injections of prostaglandins E_1 and E_2, as well as $F_1\alpha$ and $F_2\alpha$ induced fevers in sheep and rats. (Baird et al. [1974] reported that prostaglandins failed to induce a fever in the primitive mammal belonging to the monotremes, the echidna, *Tachyglossus sp.*) Studies by Feldberg and Saxena (1971) and Stitt (1973) showed that microinjections of prostaglandins into the POAH produced fevers in cats and rabbits; microinjections into other areas of the brain (posterior hypothalamus and midbrain reticular formation) failed to produce a fever.

Milton and Wendlandt were probably the first to propose that pyrogens might induce a fever via the production of specific prostaglandins and that drugs which reduce a fever (antipyretic drugs) do so by blocking the synthesis and release of prostaglandins. This seemed, at the time, to be an attractive hypothesis. For example, prostaglandins are known to be a natural constituent of the hypothalamus (Holmes and Horton 1968; Ambache et al. 1966). Also following injection of bacteria into the ventricular system, or intravenously, samples of cerebrospinal fluid contained large amounts of prostaglandinlike substances (as determined by bioassay) (Feldberg et al. 1973). Using more accurate methods of measuring the presence of prostaglandins (radioimmunoassay), Philipp-Dormston and Siegert (1974) found that following an intravenous injection of bacterial or viral pyrogens, prostaglandin E levels in the cerebrospinal fluid more than doubled. Furthermore, the well-known antipyretic drugs aspirin and indomethacin are known to be potent inhibitors of prostaglandin synthesis (Vane 1971; Smith and Willis 1971; Ferreira et al. 1971). So, (1) prostaglandins occur naturally in the hypothalamus, (2) bacterial and viral infection leads to an increase in prostaglandin levels in the cerebrospinal fluid, (3) microinjections of minute amounts of prostaglandins into the POAH lead to fevers which are indistinguishable from bacterially induced fevers, and (4) antipyretic drugs are known to inhibit prostaglandin synthesis. Unfortunately, there have also been many findings which tend to indicate that naturally occurring fevers are not prostaglandin induced.

One of the first hints that prostaglandin-induced fever might not actually be the causative agent in naturally occurring fevers came from Baird et al. (1974). These investigators reported that the primitive mammal, the echidna, would develop a fever in response to an intravenous injection of bacteria, but become hypothermic in response to an intraventricular injection of prostaglandin E_1 and E_2. Pittman et al. (1977) reported similar findings in newborn lambs. Microinjections of prostaglandins into the hypothalamus of lambs failed to produce a fever. However, if bacterial pyrogens were injected into these areas or given intravenously, a fever did occur. These results indicated that prostaglandin fevers might be dissociated from pyrogen-induced fevers.

Another interesting finding which raises a question about prostaglandin fevers is that after the lesioning of the POAH of rabbits, an intravenous injection of an endogenous pyrogen still produced a fever; however, injections of prostaglandin E_1 into the area of the lesioned POAH itself no longer produced a rise in body temperature (Veale and

Cooper 1975). The fact that injections of prostaglandins into other areas of the central nervous system failed to raise body temperature (Stitt 1973) provides further evidence that prostaglandin fevers and pyrogen-induced fevers are not the same. Lipton and Trzcinka (1976) reported somewhat opposite results. Following POAH lesions in monkeys, intraventricular infusions of prostaglandins still led to fevers. Lipton and Trzcinka suggested that these different results may be related to differences in the central nervous febrile mechanisms between these species. Since fever seems to be so conservative phylogenetically (see Chapter 3), it seems unlikely that there would be fundamental differences in the final pathway from endogenous pyrogens to the actual raising of the set-point. More likely, prostaglandin fevers simply do not share the etiology of naturally occurring fevers.

A third type of experimentally obtained information has further clouded the question of prostaglandins and fever. Because bacterial pyrogens have been shown to alter the firing rate of the temperature sensitive neurons found in the POAH (the warm-sensitive neurons decrease and the cold-sensitive neurons increase their rate of firing), one might expect that prostaglandins would lead to similar changes. Although Ford (1974) did find that microinjections of prostaglandins did excite cold-sensitive neurons in the cat, Stitt and Hardy (1975) found that this had little, if any, effect in the rabbit. Stitt and Hardy found that generally the effect of microinjections of prostaglandins was one of mild facilitation of the warm-sensitive neurons, the opposite of what one might have predicted based on work with bacterial pyrogens.

More recently, the results of a fourth type of experiment have added to the growing evidence that prostaglandins are not a component of pyrogen-induced fevers. Cranston and coworkers (1975) have shown that an intravenous infusion of an endogenous pyrogen led to a rise in rectal temperature and a rise in prostaglandin levels in the cerebrospinal fluid of rabbits (Figure 30). They then showed that an intravenous infusion of sodium salicylate, the antipyretic (and prostaglandin inhibitor), blocked the elevation in prostaglandin

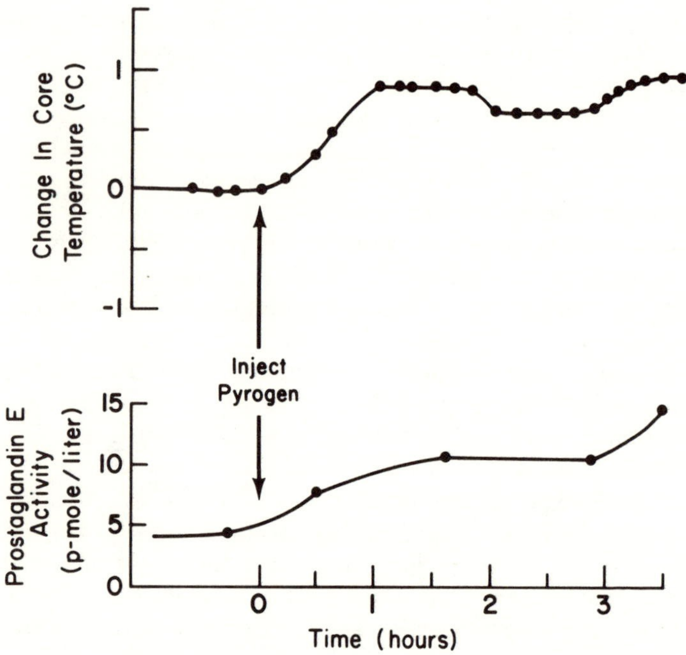

Figure 30. Responses of rabbits to an intravenous infusion of an endogenous pyrogen at time 0. Within thirty minutes, body temperature and prostaglandin E activity in the cerebrospinal fluid begins to rise. An infusion of sodium salicylate prevents this rise in cerebrospinal fluid prostaglandin E levels, but does not prevent the rise in body temperature in rabbits. (Redrawn from Cranston et al. 1975.)

levels in the cerebrospinal fluid, but not the rise in rectal temperature. They also showed that an intraventricular injection of the drug SC 19220, a potent prostaglandin antagonist, blocked prostaglandin fevers, but not fevers induced by endogenous pyrogens.

These results indicate that while there is positive evidence that prostaglandins mediate pyrogen-induced fevers, there is a growing list of doubts about the role they play in naturally occurring fevers. In an attempt to partially rescue the prostaglandins fever story, Laburn et al. (1977) have demonstrated that the precursor of prostaglandins, arachidonic acid, eventually leads to the production of two pyrogenic substances—prostaglandins and either prostaglandin endoperoxide or thromboxanes. Figure 31 shows, diagrammatically, the metabolic pathways responsible for prostaglandin production. Laburn et al. found that an intraventricular injection of the sodium salt of arachidonic acid results in a dose dependent fever in rabbits. This fever is, as predicted from Figure 31, blocked by the administration of indomethacin. However, the use of the prostaglandin antagonist SC 19220, which effectively blocks prostaglandin fevers, has little effect on fevers following injection of arachidonic acid. They concluded that either prostaglandin endoperoxide or thromboxane, or some other breakdown product or metabolite, is also pyrogenic and therefore arachidonic acid leads to the production of at least two pyrogenic substances.

Additional experiments, similar to those described above for prostaglandins, will have to be performed before a role for any of these substances in febrogenesis can be conclusively demonstrated. At present, I feel confident in stating that it is unknown whether arachidonic acid or its breakdown products have any role in naturally occurring fevers.

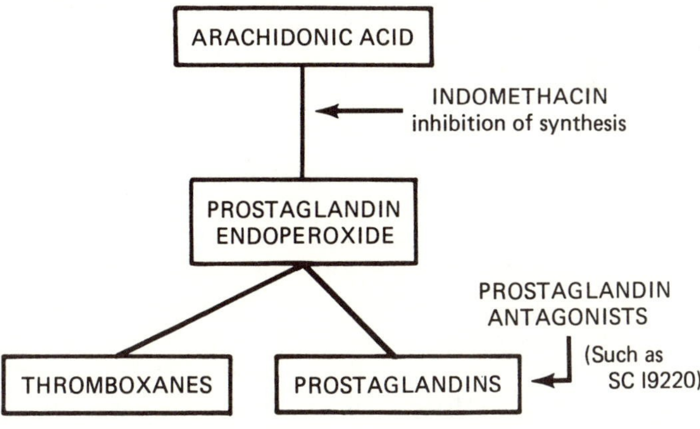

Figure 31. Diagrammatic representation of the formation of degradation products of arachidonic acid. Arrows indicate position of action of indomethacin and of antagonists of prostaglandins. (Redrawn from Hamberg et al. 1975 and from Laburn et al. 1977.)

iv. Na^+/Ca^{++} and Fever

Since the early 1900s, it has been known that the administration of various cations such as calcium (Ca^{++}) and sodium (Na^+) affects body temperature (see Sobocinska and Greenleaf 1976). There was little further experimentation on the role of these cations on thermoregulation until 1970 when Feldberg, Myers, and Veale showed that when a solution of isotonic sodium chloride was perfused through the cerebral ventricles of unanesthetized cats, a rise in body temperature resulted. When calcium was added in its normal physiological concentration to the perfusate, this rise in body temperature was blocked. From these results, Feldberg et al. suggested that these ions might play a role in maintaining the thermoregulatory set-point at a given level. These initial observations stimulated a series of experiments in many laboratories to determine the exact nature of the changes in body temperature brought about by the infusion of calcium and sodium ions.

Using a device known as a "push-pull" cannula, Myers and Veale (1970) were able to localize the effects of Na^+ and Ca^{++} on thermoregulation in the posterior hypothalamus of cats. They found that it was not the absolute levels of Na^+ or Ca^{++} which affected body temperature of these animals, but the ratio of Na^+ to Ca^{++}. When Na^+/Ca^{++} increased, body temperature increased; when Na^+/Ca^{++} decreased, body temperature decreased. The rise in body temperature caused by an increase in this ratio was accompanied by shivering, peripheral vasoconstriction, and piloerection—responses known to occur during the development of a fever (Myers and Veale 1971). The fall in body temperature caused by a decrease in this ratio was accompanied by peripheral vasodilation and a decrease in activity. Similar results have been found in rats, monkeys, and rabbits (see Myers and Buckman 1972). In the golden hamster, a mammal capable of hibernating, infusion of excess Ca^{++} led to a fall in body temperature (often approaching hibernating levels). An infusion of excess Na^+ had no effect on body temperature in these animals. Hanegan and Williams (1973) showed that an infusion of excess Ca^{++} into the POAH of another species of hibernator, the ground squirrel, also led to large drops in body temperature. Seone and Baile (1973), however, failed to find any effect of Ca^{++} infusion into the ventricular system on the body temperature of sheep.

In another type of experiment, Myers and Yaksh (1971) infused a calcium chelating agent (EGTA) into the ventricular system and posterior hypothalamus of monkeys. A chelating agent simply binds to the ion and in this case effectively removes Ca^{++} from the medium bathing the neural tissues. Infusion of EGTA either into the ventricular system or directly into the posterior hypothalamus led to rises in body temperature. Similar results have been reported using different chelating agents in cats (Clark 1971) and in dogs (Sadowski and Szczepanska-Sadowska 1974).

Body temperature can also be altered by intravenous infusions of Na^{+} and/or Ca^{++}. For example, Nielsen (1974a) has shown that the rectal temperatures of rabbits increased when hyperosmotic NaCl solution was infused into the marginal ear vein. Conversely, an infusion of $CaCl_2$ caused a fall in rectal temperature. Turlejska-Stemasiak (1974) reported that an intravenous infusion of hypertonic NaCl inhibited panting in heat stressed rabbits. These rabbits received a slow infusion of hypertonic NaCl and at the same time had their POAH warmed. In the control rabbits, respiratory rate increased by about ninety breaths per minute, whereas in four of five rabbits receiving the hypertonic NaCl, respiratory rate remained unchanged.

Greenleaf et al. (1976) found that an intravenous infusion of hypertonic NaCl had little effect on the body temperature of resting dogs; however, during exercise these dogs reached higher rectal or deep body temperatures. These results were similar to those found by Nielsen et al. (1971) for exercising human beings. In these studies, solutions of different concentrations of NaCl were drunk by the subjects. Again, body temperature did not change at rest, but during exercise body temperatures were correlated with their plasma Na^{+} concentrations. In a later study, Nielsen (1974b) also showed that when subjects drank $CaCl_2$ solutions several hours before exercise, the plateau of core temperature during exercise was lower than in control subjects. Similar results were found in exercising dogs which were given excess Ca^{++} (Sobocinska and Greenleaf 1976).

Whether these cations have a physiological role in pyrogen-induced fevers is unclear. Myers and Veale (1971) suggested that the balance between sodium and calcium could play an important part in the development of a fever due to bacterial pyrogens. They hypothesized that the ratio of Na^{+} to Ca^{++} in the posterior hypothalamus might rise during pyrogen-induced fevers. To test this hypothesis, Myers and Tytell (1972) implanted cats with a stainless steel tube over their lateral ventricles. After recovery from these surgical procedures, the brain tissue and fluid were labeled with radioactive Ca^{++} and Na^{+}. Samples of cerebrospinal fluid were periodically removed and the amounts of radioactive Ca^{++} and Na^{+} were determined. After an injection of typhoid vaccine, the amount of radioactive Ca^{++} increased and the Na^{+} decreased in the cerebrospinal fluid. The efflux of Ca^{++} into the cerebrospinal fluid paralleled the rise in body temperature of the cats. Myers and Tytell interpreted these data as indicating that since the ratio of Na^{+} to Ca^{++} in the cerebrospinal fluid fell, the ratio of Na^{+} to Ca^{++} in the hypothalamus and other central nervous areas increased, thus supporting their hypothesis that an increase in the Na^{+}/Ca^{++} had a role in the development of fever. Nielsen et al. (1973), however, found that in human beings the ratio of Na^{+} to Ca^{++} in the cerebrospinal fluid did not vary between febrile and afebrile patients. (As Nielsen et al. sampled the cerebrospinal fluid from the lumbar region, and not in the vicinity of the hypothalamus, these data might not be directly applicable to the question of whether hypothalamic cations change during fever.)

Although it is not known what specific effect changes in these cations might have on the neurons responsible for febrogenesis, the work of Hensel and Schafer (1974) has raised some interesting possibilities. Hensel and Schafer investigated the physiological effects Ca^{++} has on peripheral thermal receptors. Apparently, it has long been known that in people, an intravenous injection of Ca^{++} causes a diffuse sensation of warmth (Hirschsohn and Maendl 1922). Hensel and Schafer also point out that an intracutaneous injection of Ca^{++} was found to lower the threshold of warm sensations and to increase the threshold of cold sensations (Schreiner 1936). Hensel's and Schafer's study also found that in cats, Ca^{++} increased the firing rate of peripheral warm-sensitive neurons and decreased the firing rate of peripheral cold-sensitive neurons (Figure 32). If similar changes occurred within the central nervous areas responsible for the development of fevers, then these changes in the firing rates of neurons could account for the change in set-point during fever.

Although the theory that the ratio of Na^{+} to Ca^{++} in various regions of the brain is responsible for maintaining the

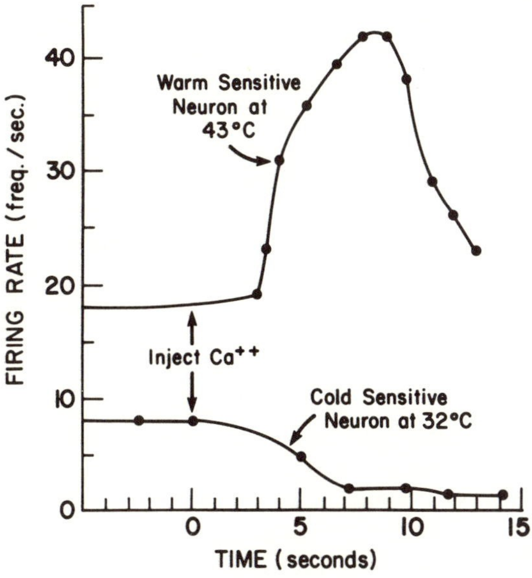

Figure 32. Discharge frequency of representative warm- and cold-sensitive neurons. Within a few seconds after adding Ca^{++} to the medium surrounding these neurons, the firing rate of the warm-sensitive neurons increased and the firing rate of the cold-sensitive neurons decreased. (Redrawn from Hensel and Schafer 1974.)

set-point at any given level seems to be fairly convincing, there are several potentially strong arguments against this theory. One of the major objections to the Na^+ to Ca^{++} ratio having a role in normal thermoregulation and fever has been that the changes in Na^+/Ca^{++} necessary to produce alterations in body temperature are generally sizeable—well above normal physiological variations. Robertshaw and Beier (1977) have noted that changes in body temperature during the human menstrual cycle might be related to changes in the *ionic* calcium levels. Almost invariably, following an infusion of excess Na^+ or Ca^{++} into the cerebrospinal fluid, or intravenously, the levels of ionic sodium or calcium are not measured. What is measured are the levels of total sodium or calcium, which includes the bound sodium and calcium as well. Although almost all sodium exists in its ionic state, this is not true for calcium (Davson 1970). As it is probably the ionic sodium or calcium that affects the temperature sensitive neurons, the measurements of the ionic concentrations of these substances are critical. Another possible explanation for why such high levels of these cations are required to produce any physiological effect might be related to the location of the neurons which are involved in febrogenesis. If the neurons are not located near the ventricles of the brain, then changing the cerebrospinal levels of Ca^{++} (or Na^+) four- or fivefold might only slightly raise the concentrations of these ions near these neurons.

Another objection to the theory that normal temperature regulation and fever are the result of changes in these ions is that the results are so variable. For example, whereas the body temperature of resting cats, rats and other rodents, rabbits, and monkeys is affected by changes in Na^+/Ca^{++}, the body temperature of resting human beings and dogs is not. It seems unlikely that the mechanism of fever should be so conservative, phylogenetically (see Chapter 3), and yet be so variable concerning the final pathway.

Before a role for Na^+/Ca^{++} in febrogenesis can be firmly established, it will be necessary to determine (1) the effects of pyrogens on the actual levels of intra- and extracellular Na^+ and Ca^{++} in the central nervous areas involved in febrogenesis, and (2) whether changing the *ionic* concentrations within these areas, by comparable values to that which occurs naturally, actually induces a fever.

v. Cyclic AMP and Fever

Many hormones and neurotransmitters, including some of those involved in thermoregulation, are thought to exert their effects via the activation or formation of cyclic 3′, 5′-adenosine monophosphate (cyclic AMP) (Milton and Dascombe 1977). Most protein hormones are insoluble in cell membranes and as a result cannot enter their target organ cells. Sutherland and his colleagues have shown that protein hormones exert their effects by binding to the cell membrane and activating an enzyme known as adenyl cyclase. The adenyl cyclase catalyzes the transformation of ATP to cyclic AMP within the cell, and it is this cyclic AMP (the "second messenger") which produces the alteration in cell function associated with that hormone (Vander et al. 1975).

There is some evidence that cyclic AMP is involved in febrogenesis. For example, injections of pyrogens have been shown to increase the levels of cyclic AMP in the cerebrospinal fluid of cats and rabbits (Milton and Dascombe 1977; Philipp-Dormston and Siegert 1975). Furthermore, using inhibitors of nucleotide phosphodiesterase, the enzyme responsible for the destruction of cyclic AMP, Dascombe (1976) has found that endotoxin-induced fever is potentiated in rabbits (but not in cats). Similar results were reported by Woolf et al. (1975) in rabbits.

The injection of cyclic AMP into several species of animals has shown that in rats and rabbits fever generally develops, whereas in cats body temperature generally falls (see Table 3). As in the case of prostaglandins and Na^{+}/Ca^{++}, it is not known whether cyclic AMP has any physiological role in pyrogen-induced fevers. Since cyclic AMP is an important second messenger for many hormones and neurotransmitters, it is likely that it does have some role in thermoregulation; however, at present this role has not been conclusively determined.

Table 3. Changes in Body Temperature by Central Nervous System Administration of Cyclic AMP (based on Willies et al. 1976)

Species	*Site of Injection*	*Response*
Rat	Hypothalamus	Body temperature rose
Cat	Lateral ventricle and hypothalamus	Body temperature generally fell
Rabbit	Lateral ventricle and POAH	Body temperature generally rose

vi. Antipyretic Drugs

In large doses, antipyretic drugs such as sodium salicylate, indomethacin, acetophenetidin, and paracetamol produce hypothermia in afebrile experimental animals (Satinoff 1972; Yokoi 1969; Clark and Cumby 1975; Clark 1970). The hypothermic effects of these drugs appear to be most pronounced when the animals are in a low environmental temperature. The dose required to produce effective antipyresis in febrile experimental animals is generally considerably less than that required to produce hypothermia in afebrile animals.

There is some controversy over the central vs. peripheral effects of antipyretic drugs. Gander et al. (1967) suggested that antipyretic drugs such as sodium salicylate induce antipyresis by inhibiting the synthesis and/or release of endogenous pyrogens. They found that salicylates reduced the yield of endogenous pyrogens from white blood cells obtained from rabbits. As a result of these findings, they concluded that in rabbits, the antipyretic effect of salicylates is not within the central nervous system but rather is peripheral, acting on the leukocytes to inhibit the formation and/or release of endogenous pyrogens.

Many other investigators have found just the opposite results. For example, Adler et al. (1969) reported that in human beings, a steady state fever could be produced by giving an intravenous priming injection of an endogenous pyrogen followed by a continuous infusion of the endogenous pyrogen. When sodium salicylate was given to these subjects, the fever decreased. If antipyretic drugs worked solely by inhibiting the production and/or release of endogenous pyrogens, then these drugs should not have produced antipyresis in these subjects. Similar results were found in rabbits (Cranston et al. 1970).

Clark and Moyer (1972) found that the antipyretic drugs acetaminophen and sodium salicylate had no effect on the release of the endogenous pyrogen from cat leukocytes obtained from activated blood or from peritoneal exudates. Clark and Cumby (1975) reported similar results for the antipyretic drug indomethacin. Furthermore, van Miert et al. (1972) demonstrated that sodium salicylate did not block the release of endogenous pyrogens in white blood cells from goats or from rabbits. Also, Hoo et al. (1972) reported that the drug acetylsalicylic acid (aspirin) had no effect on the production of endogenous pyrogens by rabbit white blood cells. Lastly, Bodel et al. (1973) found that incubation of human blood leukocytes with high concentrations of salicylates had no effect on their capacity to release an endogenous pyrogen.

No satisfactory explanation has been given for the discrepancy between the results obtained by Gander's group and those obtained by other laboratories. It is apparent that whereas antipyretic drugs may have some peripheral effect, their primary action occurs centrally.

The mode of action of these antipyretic drugs has not yet been established. Recall that antipyretic drugs have been shown to alter the firing rate of temperature sensitive neurons located within the POAH. Studies by Wit and Wang (1968) and later bv Schoener and Wang (1975) have shown that microinjections of sodium acetylsalicylate into the POAH had little effect on the neuronal discharge of temperature sensitive neurons in afebrile cats. However, during pyrogen-induced fever, the microinjection of this antipyretic drug returned these temperature sensitive neurons back toward their original firing rate. If these neurons are actually involved in febrogenesis, then the effects of sodium acetylsalicylate on these neurons could explain the mode of action of antipyretic drugs. How antipyretic drugs actually cause these changes in neuronal firing rates is unknown. If elevations in the concentration of prostaglandins play a role in febrogenesis, then the mechanism of action of antipyretic drugs could be explained by their inhibition of prostaglandin synthesis. However, as described earlier, a definitive role for prostaglandins in fever has not been established. Furthermore, the results of Stitt's and Hardy's work (1975) have shown that prostaglandins do not alter the firing rate of temperature sensitive neurons in the POAH. Therefore, while it appears that antipyretic drugs exert most of their effects centrally, it is still unclear what mechanism is responsible for their mode of action.

Summary

Careful studies on the biology of fever were not possible until the development of accurate temperature measuring instruments in the eighteenth century. By the late 1800s, Liebermeister had determined experimentally that during fever a person *regulated* his body temperature at an elevated level. As a result, conditions such as hypothermia and hyperthermia could be distinguished from fever.

Many substances serve as activators, or initiators, of the febrile response. Whether these activators are endotoxins from Gram-negative bacteria, Gram-positive bacteria, viruses, or other types of antigens, they all seem to produce a fever via the production of endogenous pyrogens from the host's own immunologically active phagocytic cells such as granulocytes, monocytes, macrophages, and Kupffer cells. Endogenous pyrogens apparently affect the thermoregulatory areas of the central nervous system in the region of the POAH, the brainstem, and perhaps other areas. The precise mechanism behind endogenous pyrogens' effect on the thermoregulatory set-point is unknown.

Results from many laboratories have implicated prostaglandins, the Na^+ to Ca^{++} ratio, and cyclic AMP in the pathway from endogenous pyrogens to the elevation in set-point. There are convincing arguments both in favor of and against the role each of these substances has in febrogenesis. At present, it is unknown whether any of these chemicals has any role in the development of pyrogen-induced fever. Lastly, the effect of antipyretic drugs appears to be primarily one which affects the central nervous area or areas responsible for the elevation in set-point. The precise mechanism of action of these drugs is unknown.

3. The Evolution of Fever

Introduction

A careful description of the phylogeny of fever would be very helpful to an understanding of many of its fundamental characteristics. It might also provide animal models which could be used to answer the question of whether fever was an adaptive mechanism which aided the host organism in combating infection (see Chapter 4). As a result, in 1973 a series of investigations was initiated to characterize the febrile responses of the vertebrates.

The Evolution of the Vertebrates

In order to trace the phylogeny of fever in the vertebrates, it is first necessary to have a fundamental understanding of the evolutionary relationships of the vertebrates. There are approximately 46 thousand different species of living vertebrates. This is a small group of organisms compared to many others. For example, there are about 750 thousand species of insects, and an estimated 500 thousand species of round worms or nematodes. The Vertebrata constitute one of three subphyla in the phylum Chordata (the other two being the Urochordata [tunicates and sea squirts], and the Cephalochordata [the lancelets]). The vertebrates are, as their name implies, characterized by the possession of a backbone composed of a series of vertebrae. There are seven classes of living vertebrates—Agnatha (lampreys and hagfishes), Chondrichthyes (sharks, skates, rays, etc.), Osteichthyes (bony fishes), Amphibia (frogs, salamanders, etc.), Reptilia (snakes, lizards, turtles, crocodiles, etc.), Aves (birds), and Mammalia (monotremes, marsupials, and placentals).

The earliest known vertebrates, the Agnatha, appeared in

the Ordovician period, approximately 4 to 5 hundred million years ago (Figure 33). The remarkable feature about the placoderms was their possession of jaws. The noted paleontologist Edwin Colbert (1961) has called the appearance of jaws one of the "great revolutions in the history of the vertebrates." Jawless vertebrates are restricted to fairly narrow niches. They can evolve as filter feeders, sucking small organisms and dead organic materials into their pharynx and straining out the water by their gills, or as in the case of the present-day jawless vertebrates (the lampreys and hagfishes), as parasites. The presence of jaws permitted the vertebrates to acquire a considerably wider variety of food sources than was available to their jawless ancestors and was largely responsible for the eventual radiation of the vertebrates onto the land (Blair et al. 1957).

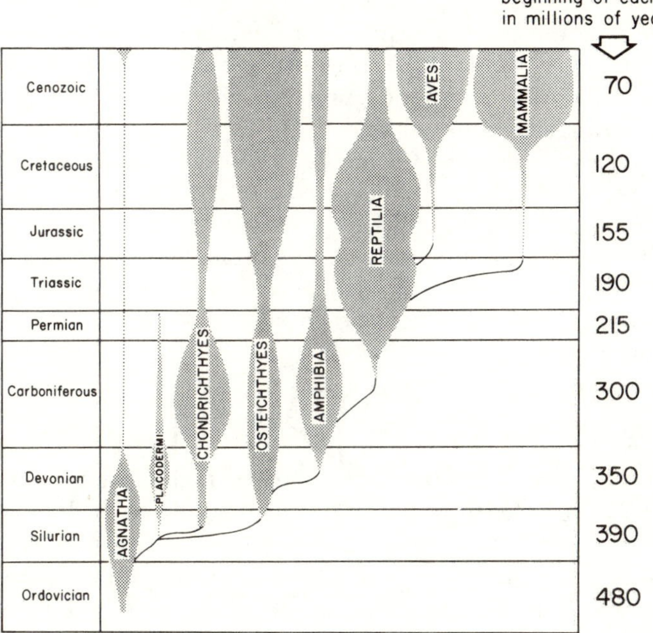

Figure 33. The evolution of the vertebrate classes. (Based on Romer 1966.)

The Chondrichthyes and Osteichthyes evolved from the Placodermi. The Chondrichthyes, unlike the Osteichthyes, are not in the main line of evolution to the terrestrial vertebrates. The Osteichthyes, or bony fishes, radiated into two main groups—the ray finned fishes and the lobe finned or air breathing fishes (Colbert 1961). This latter group of fishes consists of two orders—the lungfishes or dipnoans, and the crossopterygians. Several species of lungfishes and one species of crossopterygian, the coelocanth (*Latimeria sp.*), survive to this day. It was a relative of the coelocanth that gave rise to the first Amphibia in the late Devonian period, some 320 million years ago. The transition from the aquatic environment to the semiterrestrial existence of these early amphibians afforded them many advantages. For example, new sources of food and shelter became immediately available. Further, in times of drought, the amphibians could now move from one pond to another in search of water. Although amphibians can spend considerable periods of time on land, they were (and are) drawn to water to reproduce. Amphibian eggs are poorly protected and would soon dry out or dessicate if left on land.

By the middle of the Carboniferous period, some 280 million years ago, the Reptilia evolved from the Amphibia. The great advantage reptiles had, compared to amphibians, was the possession of an egg which was protected from dessication by a hard exterior or shell, and the presence of a fluid-filled sac or amnion which bathed the developing embryo in its own aquatic environment. The presence of this "amniote egg" completely freed terrestrial vertebrates from their dependence upon habitable water during some stage of their development.

The evolution of birds from their reptilian ancestors has recently received a great deal of attention. According to Bakker and Galton (1974), birds and dinosaurs should be grouped together into one class, the Dinosauria, which diverged from the lines of reptiles which led to the surviving reptilian species in the Triassic period about 180 million years ago.

Although mammals did not appear until perhaps 175 million years ago, the group of reptiles which gave rise to the Mammalia (the therapsids) diverged from the main line of reptilian evolution in the Permian period, about 200 million years ago.

The advantage birds and mammals had over other classes of vertebrates was their ability to produce significant amounts of heat internally (endothermy). Although this trait is not unique to birds and mammals (see Chapter 1), other groups of vertebrates have only a few scattered examples of endothermy (the possible exception to this might be the dinosaurs which, as Bakker [1975] and others have hypothesized, were also endothermic). Endothermy allows the organism to remain active during periods of cool weather, whether this occurs daily or seasonally.

From this brief summary of the highlights of vertebrate evolution, one can see that the different vertebrate classes have been separated by hundreds of millions of years. Several points are worth stressing. The first of these is that in physiological studies of a comparative nature, one is usually comparing present-day representatives of these vertebrate classes. Based on similarities in, for example, the endocrine or nervous system, one often makes hypotheses that these similarities indicate a long phylogenetic history for that trait. For example, in studying the phylogeny of a specific hormone (hormone X), one might find that this hormone is present in all living groups of vertebrates, excluding the Agnatha and the Chondrichthyes. As a result, one might hypothesize that this hormone evolved after the divergence of the bony fishes from the Chondrichthyes, sometime in the middle Silurian period, about 400 million years ago (hypothesis 1). There are two alternate hypotheses. One is that the Agnatha and Chondrichthyes also had hormone X but that selective pressures were such that this hormone was lost (hypothesis 2). If hypothesis 2 were true, then the phylogeny of hormone X would be even older than 400 million years. Another possibility is that the bony fishes, amphibians, reptiles, birds, and mammals, all independently, and perhaps recently, evolved this hormone (hypothesis 3). The chances of five classes of vertebrates, each consisting of thousands of species, independently evolving essentially the same hormone (or any other substance) is highly unlikely. Although the exact phylogeny of hormone X will never be known, the most reasonable hypotheses are numbers 1 or 2.

Another point worth noting is that it is remarkable that even though the vertebrate classes are separated from each other by long spans of time, so many features of their anatomy and physiology have remained similar. It is generally true that the longer a group of organisms has been phylogenetically separated from each other, the more dissimilar they become. (This is why different species of mammals, for example, which might be separated by only 70 million years or so, are generally more similar than is a species of mammal to a species of bird, which might be separated by 250 million years.) The presence of those traits which remain phylogenetically conservative argues for the adaptive or beneficial nature of that particular anatomical or physiological characteristic.

Why Should Fever Have a Long Evolutionary History?

In Chapter 1, thermoregulation was partitioned into the three components of the reflex arc—sensors, integrators, and effectors (see Figure 11). A comparison of these three limbs of the reflex arc in vertebrates from the bony fishes through the mammals indicated that the sensation and integration of body temperature in these groups were similar (see Table 1). The primary distinction between the endothermic and ectothermic vertebrates was that the endotherms possessed effectors which would allow them to generate sufficient heat to raise their body temperature significantly above the environmental temperature. Other effector mechanisms (regional control over blood flow, various means of evaporating water, and various behavioral responses) were found in several vertebrate classes, and the presence of these effectors could not be predicted based on whether the organism was endothermic or ectothermic.

In Chapter 2, the biology of fever was extensively discussed. It is believed that endogenous pyrogens, by some as yet unknown mechanism, trigger a rise in the organism's set-point. The organism then employs physiological and/or behavioral means to elevate its body temperature to this raised set-point. From extensive investigations, it is clear that pyrogens affect either the sensory or integrating limb of the thermoregulatory reflex. Since these are the two limbs of the reflex which are so phylogenetically conservative, it seems reasonable to hypothesize that all these classes of vertebrates would respond to appropriate activators by developing a fever.

Fever in the Vertebrates

A. Mammals

A random selection of 100 research articles involving some aspect of the biology of fever reveals that the laboratory rabbit is the most commonly used experimental animal for these types of studies (see Table 4).

Most of the mammals listed in Table 4 are commonly used laboratory animals (the possible exceptions being sheep, goats, and certainly the echidna). All developed fevers in response to an injection with the appropriate activator.

There has been little comparative research on the febrile responses of mammals. Whereas veterinary textbooks often include the normal body temperatures of the larger domes-

Table 4. Animals Used in Fever Research (based on 100 randomly selected articles)

Animal	*Number of Papers*
Laboratory rabbit	54
Cat	16
Laboratory rat	8
Dog	6
Rhesus monkey	4
Squirrel monkey	4
Sheep (and lamb)	3
Guinea pig	3
Goat	1
Echidna	1
	n = 100

ticated animals, as well as those of some of the larger animals found in zoos (elephants, lions, etc.), there are little experimental data on the responses of these animals to injections of endotoxins, viruses, endogenous pyrogens, etc. The discussion of the febrile responses of the mammals will be brief, because much of this material was covered in detail in Chapter 2.

a. *Activators of Fever*. Mammals develop fever in response to injections of Gram-negative bacteria (containing endotoxins), Gram-positive bacteria, viruses, antigens resulting in hypersensitivity reactions, and to certain types of malignant tumors. Excluding human beings, virtually all of this research has been performed on the laboratory rabbit and cat.

b. *Endogenous Pyrogens*. Heat sensitive pyrogenic proteins have been isolated from many species of mammals including the rabbit, dog, cat, goat, guinea pig, and human being. Apparently, all of the above activators of fever work via the production of endogenous pyrogens which are produced by the host's own phagocytic cells such as polymorphonuclear granulocytes, monocytes, macrophages, and Kupffer cells. (Most of this latter information has been obtained using the laboratory rabbit.)

c. *Fever and the Central Nervous System*. During a fever, the mammal acts as though its thermoregulatory set-point has been elevated. As a result, the febrile organism employs both physiological and behavioral effector mechanisms in order to raise and maintain its body temperature at this elevated level. From data obtained largely from the laboratory rabbit, it appears that endogenous pyrogens exert their effects on the central nervous system, ultimately resulting in this elevation in set-point. The intermediate messengers between endogenous pyrogens and the rise in the set-point are unknown.

Prostaglandins (particularly those of the E series) produce fevers when injected into the brains of many species of mammals. As a result of this and related observations, prostaglandins have been implicated in febrogenesis. There are, as described in Chapter 2, serious objections to prostaglandins having a role in naturally occurring fevers.

Another proposed intermediary between endogenous pyrogens and the elevated set-point is the ratio of sodium to calcium ions. When this ratio is experimentally raised, a fever develops in some species of mammals. There are, however, several objections to the Na^{+}/Ca^{++} having a role in naturally occurring fevers. Cyclic AMP is another proposed intermediary in the pathway leading to the elevation in set-point. As in the case of prostaglandins and the Na^{+}/Ca^{++}, there are also serious objections to cyclic AMP having a role in naturally occurring fevers.

Lastly, antipyretic drugs such as sodium salicylate, indomethacin, acetaminophen, etc. have all been shown to reduce fevers in mammals. Most evidence indicates that these drugs work on the central nervous system, resulting in the return of the set-point toward normal. Until a few years ago, these drugs were thought to work by inhibiting prostaglandin synthesis. The exact mechanism of action of these drugs (in light of the current controversy over prostaglandins and fever) is unknown.

At the risk of being repetitious, most of what we know about the febrile responses of mammals is based on work involving only two or three species. A need exists for more comparative observations in order to be able to make some general statements concerning the activators of fever, the production of endogenous pyrogens, and the biochemical pathways leading to the elevation in the thermoregulatory set-point.

B. Birds

Little is known about the febrile responses of birds. In many clinical studies, the temperature of diseased birds has been measured by inserting a thermometer into the bird's rectum (or cloaca). This technique for measuring the body temperature of animals (particularly small endotherms) often leads to spurious results since these animals can, and often do, raise their core temperature 1° or 2°C within a few minutes of handling. More careful temperature data have been obtained from birds which have had their body temperature continuously recorded over a period ranging from several hours to several days. This has been accomplished by using temperature sensitive probes which have been taped or sutured in place, or by using telemetry (small, wireless, thermally sensitive devices which transmit temperature via radio frequencies). The results of this handful of papers on the avian febrile response are summarized below.

a. *Activators of Fever*. In 1968, van Miert and Frens reported that injections of endotoxins isolated from *E. coli* bacteria led to a fever in chickens. These fevers averaged about 0.6°C and peaked about three hours after the injection. Pittman et al. (1976) reported that they were unable to induce fevers in chickens following injections of endotoxins isolated from the bacterium *Salmonella abortus equi*. Using doses comparable to those used by van Miert and Frens, they found that at the higher doses, the body temperature of their birds fell during the second hour following the injection. These experiments were terminated at the end of three hours.

In 1975, we reported the results of our investigations on the febrile response of pigeons (D'Alecy and Kluger 1975). In these investigations, we used the bacterium *Pasteurella multocida*, a common avian pathogen. Since there had been few reports concerning the febrile response of birds, we continuously monitored the body temperature of these animals for periods of up to one week. The results of injections of alcohol-killed bacteria are summarized in Figures 34 and 35. Injections of the low doses of dead bacteria led to fevers after a latency of about three hours. The injection of the higher doses of dead bacteria led to a statistically significant fall in body temperature similar to that observed by Pittman et al. (1976). This fall in body temperature was then followed by a series of oscillations in body temperature. Depending on the dose, a fever then developed within five to ten hours following the injection. It is currently unknown what caused the initial fall and subsequent series of oscillations in body temperature.

Injections of pigeons with live bacteria lead to long-lasting fevers (Figure 36). Following an injection of live bacteria, the pigeons develop a fever within the first three to four hours

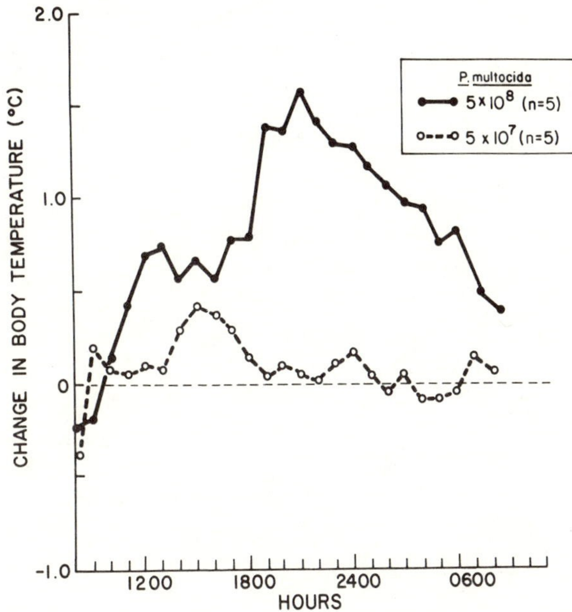

Figure 34. Average changes in pigeon body temperature in response to injection of dead bacteria (*Pasteurella multocida*) at 0800 hr. (1 ml of $5 \times 10^7 - 5 \times 10^8$). Injection of 5×10^7 organisms led to little elevation in body temperature. Injection of 5×10^8 led to an average fever of 0.80°C. (From D'Alecy and Kluger 1975.)

and maintain this fever for several days, until they either recover from the infection or die. Oftentimes, just prior to death, their body temperature rises sharply to as high as 45°C.

To my knowledge, there have been no carefully controlled studies concerning the thermal effects induced by other activators in birds (e.g. Gram-positive bacteria, viruses, etc.).

b. *Endogenous Pyrogens*. It is not presently known whether endogenous pyrogens can be isolated from the immunologically active phagocytic cells of birds. However, since both mammals and reptiles have been shown to produce heat labile proteins, endogenous pyrogens, in response to ac-

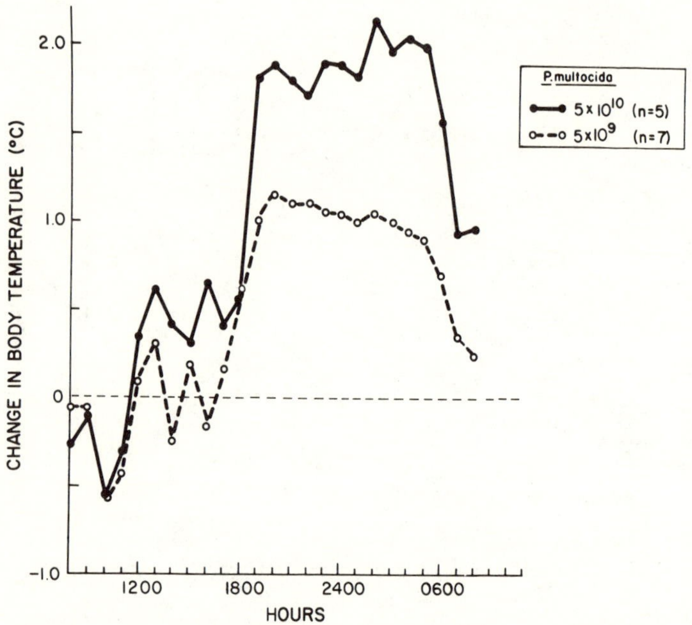

Figure 35. Average changes in pigeon body temperature in response to injection of dead bacteria (*Pasteurella multocida*) at 0800 hr. (1 ml of $5 \times 10^9 - 5 \times 10^{10}$). Injection of these higher doses of bacteria led to an initial decline in body temperature followed by a series of oscillations and then ultimately to fevers averaging 0.50° and 1.06°C respectively. (From D'Alecy and Kluger 1975.)

tivators of fever, it is likely that birds (which also evolved from reptiles) will eventually be shown to produce these substances.

c. *Fever and the Central Nervous System*. Febrile birds generally elevate their body temperature by using those behavioral and physiological responses which decrease heat loss and increase heat gain from the environment, and by increasing their metabolic heat production. These responses are, as in all vertebrates, coordinated by the central nervous system.

Assuming that birds produce and release endogenous pyrogens in response to the appropriate activators of fever, the next question is, as in mammals, what are the inter-

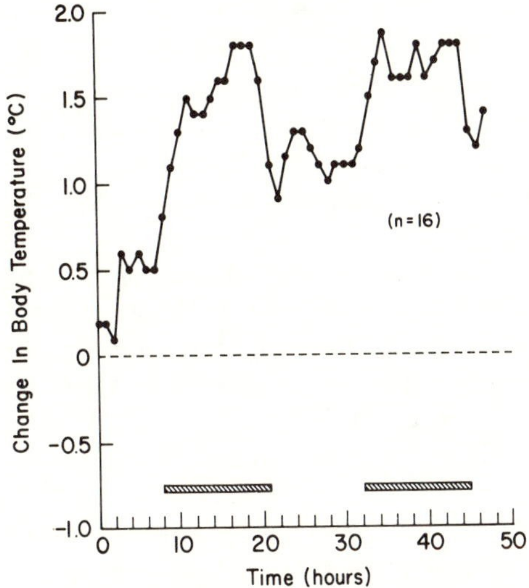

Figure 36. Average changes in pigeon body temperature in response to infection with live bacteria (*Pasteurella multocida*) (1 ml of 1 x 10^8 bacteria). Following the injection of live bacteria, a fever developed within a few hours and lasted for several days. Note that the magnitude of the fever varies with the time of day. (Striped bars indicate periods of darkness.)

mediary messengers in the pathway from endogenous pyrogens to an elevated set-point? Several investigators have shown that an injection of prostaglandin E_1 into the hypothalamus of chickens induces a dose dependent rise in body temperature (Nistico and Marley 1973; Artunkal and Marley 1974; Pittman et al. 1976). Injections of low doses of prostaglandin into other regions of the brain failed to produce a fever. As in mammals, it is not known whether prostaglandin-induced fevers have any relationship to naturally occurring fevers.

The effects of intrahypothalamic injections of Na^+ or Ca^{++}, and cyclic AMP on the thermal responses of birds are, to my knowledge, unknown. Oral administration of the antipyretic drugs acetylsalicylic acid or sodium salicylate led to the attenuation of bacterial fevers in both pigeons and chickens (D'Alecy and Kluger 1975; Pittman et al. 1976).

To summarize, these results demonstrate that birds do develop fevers in response to bacterial infection. These fevers often take considerably longer to develop than fevers in mammals (see Figure 24). The reason for this longer latency might be related to the time necessary to produce and release sufficient quantities of endogenous pyrogens.

Little is known about the thermal responses of birds to activators of fever other than Gram-negative bacteria or their endotoxins. Less is known about the effects of Na^{+}/Ca^{++} and cyclic AMP on the body temperature of birds. Lastly, antipyretic drugs can reduce the fever produced by dead Gram-negative bacteria or their endotoxins.

C. Reptiles

Much has been written about reptilian thermoregulation (see, for example, the excellent review by Templeton 1970). Most reptiles will regulate their body temperature to varying degrees. Since most living reptiles are ectotherms, this regulation of body temperature is achieved largely by behavioral responses. Subtle changes in their body posture or color can lead to marked changes in the rate of heat transfer (by conduction, convection, or radiation) between their bodies and the environment.

The most carefully investigated group of reptiles are those that rely directly on solar thermal energy to raise their body temperature—the "heliothermic" reptiles. Heliotherms, such as snakes, lizards, and crocodiles, generally begin their activity period in the morning by basking in the sunlight to raise their body temperature. Like heliothermic insects (see Figure 9), these reptiles often orient themselves in such a manner as to maximize their rate of warm-up. Once their body temperature has reached the "preferred" or active level, the reptiles will alter their angle of orientation toward the sun, move into the shade, or perform other behavioral (and to a lesser extent physiological) responses which maintain their body temperature at a fairly constant level.

A key point about thermoregulation in reptiles is that in

their natural environment (where the environmental temperature can vary more than 30°C between day and night) this is an *active* process. In order to maintain a fairly narrow body temperature in the natural environment, these animals must either shuttle between the shade and sunlight, elicit subtle or gross changes in their body posture, or employ other behavioral and/or physiological responses to regulate their body temperature.

To investigate the effects of various pyrogens, drugs, etc., on the body temperature of a reptile, one must simulate (to a certain extent) its natural environment. For example, if the environmental temperature were maintained at a constant level (as occurs in most laboratories), clearly the reptile could not select a higher or lower temperature, and therefore its body temperature would soon be approximately equal to the environmental temperature.

To study the febrile responses of reptiles, we selected two species of lizards which were known (from prior studies) to regulate their body temperature within fairly narrow ranges—the desert iguana (*Dipsosaurus dorsalis*) and the green iguana (*Iguana iguana*). Initially we tested the thermal responses of reptiles in a shuttle box which was heated at one end to above the preferred body temperature of these animals, and cooled at the other end to below their preferred temperatures (see Figure 22 [A]). In later studies, we tested these animals in a simulated desert environment (Figure 37). This chamber had an area of two square meters and was covered on the botton with about 10 to 15 cm of sand. The lights were on a twelve-hour-light and twelve-hour-dark cycle. During the day the room temperature was controlled to about 30°C for the experiments with the desert iguanas and to about 25°C for the experiments with the green iguanas. At night, the environmental temperature fell. Suspended above the chamber were heat lamps which were timed to go on and off at different times during the day. As a result, the sand temperature beneath these heat lamps (when they were on) would reach a temperature as high as 50° to 55°C. Therefore, during the day, the desert

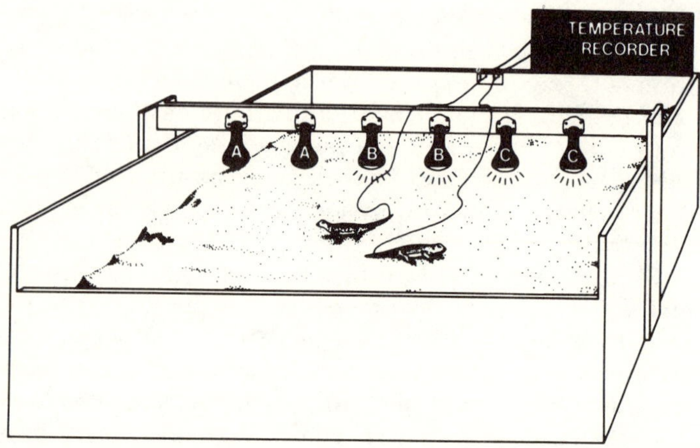

Figure 37. Experimental desert environment used to study thermal responses of lizards. The chamber was placed in a temperature control room where the environmental temperature could be controlled at different temperatures during the day and night. Fluorescent lights were on a twelve-hour light and twelve-hour dark cycle. Heat lamps labeled A were on from 0600 to 1000 hr., those labeled B were on from 0900 to 1500 hr., and those labeled C were on from 1000 to 1800 hr. Areas directly beneath these heat lamps reached temperatures of about 50°C during the on hours, allowing each lizard to select an ambient temperature from room temperature to close to 50°C. (From Bernheim and Kluger 1976a.)

iguanas could select an environmental temperature ranging between 30° and 55°C, and the green iguanas between 25° and 50°C.

a. *Activators of Fever*. To date, we have investigated the febrile responses of two species of reptiles, the desert and green iguanas. These species develop fevers in response to an injection of various species of bacteria (*Aeromonas hydrophila, Pasteurella hemolytica*, and *Citrobacter diversus*) (Figure 38). These bacteria were selected since they are all known to be reptilian pathogens.

Following injection with these bacteria, fevers generally developed within three to four hours, and often lasted for several days. During this time, the lizards would (if given the opportunity) select a higher environmental temperature,

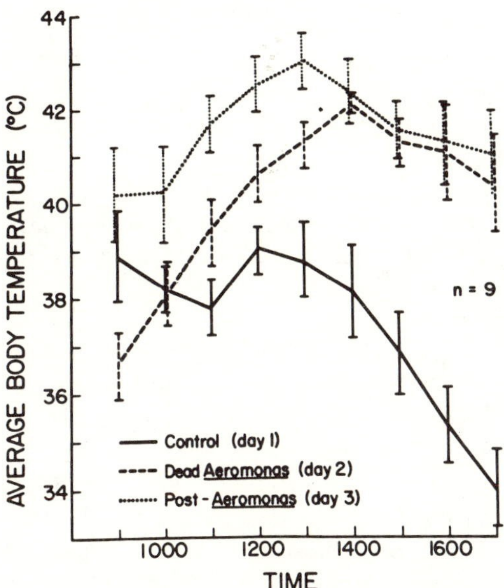

Figure 38. Changes in the body temperatuares of nine desert iguanas after injection with dead *Aeromonas hydrophila* (4 x 10^9 organisms) on body temperature (mean hourly body temperature ± 1 SE). On control days (day 1), lizards had a mean body temperature of about 38°C. Following inoculation with dead bacteria (day 2) they selected a warmer environment and as a result their body temperature rose to ca. 42°C within about five hours. This elevated body temperature persisted through the following day (day 3). (From Bernheim and Kluger 1976a.)

and as a result, their body temperature would become elevated above their afebrile (or control) levels. When these lizards were placed in a constant temperature chamber they were not able to raise their body temperatures, and as a result their body temperatures did not rise following the injections with bacteria. Clearly, these lizards were behaving as though their thermoregulatory set-point had become elevated (i.e. febrile), and as a result they actively sought out higher environmental temperatures leading to an elevation in their body temperature.

It is not currently known whether other species of reptiles also develop fevers in response to bacterial infection. We would, however, predict that since the only species of reptiles that were studied developed fevers in response to infection, it is likely that other species of thermoregulating reptiles would also develop fevers following inoculation with the appropriate pathogens.

It is also unknown whether reptiles develop fevers in response to activators of fever other than Gram-negative bacteria. Again, we would predict that various agents which induce inflammatory reactions, infections, etc., would also probably induce fevers.

b. *Endogenous Pyrogens*. Leukocytes obtained from peritoneal exudates of desert iguanas produce an endogenous pyrogenlike substance (Bernheim and Kluger 1977). Injecting this substance into lizards resulted in their developing a fever with a latency of about three to four hours and a duration of about five hours (Figure 39). Denaturation (by heating to about 80°C) resulted in the complete loss of this pyrogenicity. It is likely that in reptiles (as is thought to occur in mammals), the various activators induce fevers by producing heat sensitive proteins, endogenous pyrogens.

To test whether an endogenous pyrogen has cross-class reactivity (that is, induces a fever when injected into another species from a different class of organisms), an endogenous pyrogen was isolated from rabbit peritoneal exudates and injected into desert iguanas. These lizards developed fevers which, for some unknown reason, lasted longer than two days. The opposite experiment, injecting an endogenous pyrogen from lizards into rabbits, has not yet been done since it is likely that this would require white blood cells from dozens of lizards (each weighing about 40 grams) to produce an adequate dose of an endogenous pyrogen to produce a fever in a mammal the size of the laboratory rabbit.

c. *Fever and the Central Nervous System*. Since lizards raise their body temperature almost entirely by behavioral means, pyrogens must be acting on the central nervous system to elevate the thermoregulatory set-point. The intermediaries between the endogenous pyrogen and this elevation in set-point are unknown.

It is, however, known that the antipyretic drug, sodium

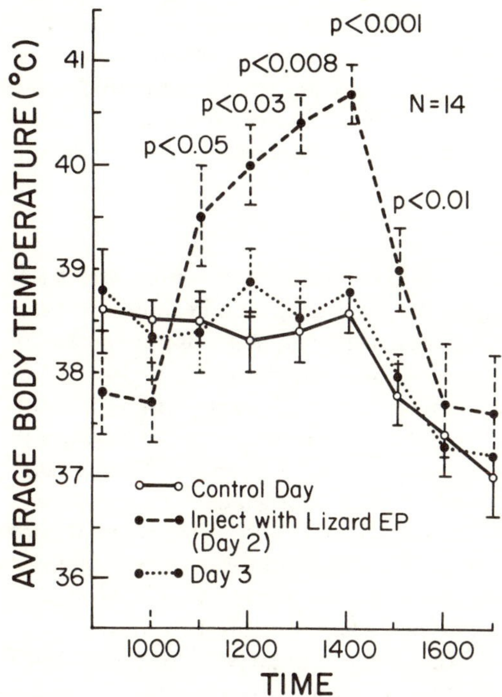

Figure 39. Effects of injection of lizard endogenous pyrogen on the mean hourly body temperature (± SE) of fourteen desert iguanas. The injection was made at about 0900 hr. on day 2. A fever developed with a latency of about three to four hours and lasted about five hours. (From Bernheim and Kluger 1977.)

salicylate, will lead to effective antipyresis (Bernheim and Kluger 1976a). Whether desert iguanas were injected with dead or live bacteria, administration of the appropriate dose of sodium salicylate led to their selection of a cooler environment and thereafter their body temperature remained at the control or afebrile levels.

To summarize, lizards develop fevers in response to injections of various species of Gram-negative bacteria. It is believed that the various activators of fever in reptiles induce the production of an endogenous pyrogen from the host's own leukocytes and perhaps from other phagocytic cells.

How the endogenous pyrogen eventually leads to an elevation in set-point is currently unknown. In any event, the febrile lizard actively raises its body temperature and regulates around a new higher level. Lastly, sodium salicylate is an effective antipyretic drug during bacterial infection in lizards.

D. Amphibians

Amphibians tend to regulate their body temperature less precisely than reptiles (Brattstrom 1970). Perhaps the most likely explanation for their relatively poor ability to control their body temperature within narrow limits is that in terrestrial or semiterrestrial amphibians the precise regulation of body temperature would lead to problems related to salt and water balance. Amphibians often have a moist skin which is used for, among other things, exchanges of gases (respiration). Water is lost via evaporation from the skin of amphibians more easily than from the tough scaly skin of reptiles, or from the feathered or furred skin of birds and mammals. To regulate body temperature to within a fairly narrow range would often result in large amounts of water being lost, which would lead to an increase in the concentration of salts and other solutes. As a result, selection pressures have likely resulted in some compromise between the regulation of body temperature and of salt and water.

Many amphibians, nevertheless, still regulate their body temperature. As in reptiles, most of this regulation tends to be by behavior—the selection of a warmer or cooler microhabitat. The thermal responses of many of these ectotherms have been extensively studied and are reviewed by Brattstrom (1970).

To determine whether amphibians develop fevers in response to infection, a terrestrial species, the green tree frog (*Hyla cinerea*), and two aquatic species, the leopard frog (*Rana pipiens*) and bullfrog (*Rana catesbeiana*) tadpoles (larvae of frogs) were injected with *A. hydrophila* and their thermal responses recorded. In addition, a third species of aquatic amphibian, the frog *Rana esculenta*, has been injected with various species of killed Mycobacteria. The green tree frogs were provided with a heat source in one area of their cage and were allowed to select their preferred thermal microclimate. The tadpoles were allowed to select their preferred body temperature by swimming between two chambers of different temperatures. The *Rana esculenta* were placed in a thermal gradient where they were allowed to select their preferred body temperature. The results of these studies are described below.

a. *Activators of Fever*. Both tree frogs and tadpoles responded to an injection of *A. hydrophila* by developing a fever (Kluger 1977; Casterlin and Reynolds 1977a). These fevers were the result of their actively selecting a warmer microclimate. When prevented from selecting this warmer environment, their body temperatures remained at the control levels. In all cases, the average fevers were over 2°C above the control or afebrile levels (Figure 40). *R. esculenta* also responded to injections of bacteria by developing a fever (Myhre et al. 1977). It is not known whether other activators will induce fevers in amphibians.

b. *Endogenous Pyrogens*. Myhre et al. (1977) have obtained preliminary evidence that the blood of injected frogs produces an endogenous pyrogenlike substance which leads to fevers of short latency.

c. *Fever and the Central Nervous System*. Clearly, fevers in amphibians are, as in other vertebrates, the result of an elevation in the thermoregulatory set-point. While it is not known how this comes about, Myhre et al. (1977) have shown that injections of prostaglandin E_1 into the diencephalon of frogs led to fevers of short latency.

E. Fishes

Fishes also regulate their body temperature by selecting different thermal environments. To study the febrile responses of fishes, Reynolds and his coworkers designed a shuttle chamber which allowed the fish to select their preferred body temperature. To date, they have reported the results of their investigations on the febrile responses of

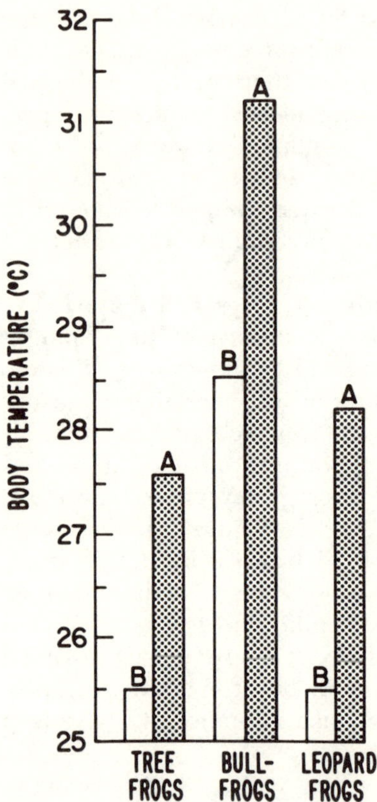

Figure 40. Average body temperature of treefrogs, bullfrog tadpoles, and leopard frog tadpoles before (B) and after (A) injection with dead bacteria (*Aeromonas hydrophila*). (Based on Kluger 1977 and Casterlin and Reynolds 1977a.)

bluegill sunfish (*Lepomis macrochirus*), largemouth bass (*Micropterus salmoides*), and goldfish (*Carassius auratus*). The results of these studies are described below.

a. *Activators of Fever*. Injections of bluegill sunfish, largemouth bass, and goldfish with *A. hydrophila* led to fevers of 2° to 3°C (Reynolds et al. 1976; Reynolds 1977; Reynolds and Covert 1977). Reynolds and coworkers have also shown that injections of other activators, such as the Gram-positive bacterium *Staphylococcus aureus* also cause fevers in freshwater fishes (Reynolds et al. 1978a, b).

b. *Endogenous Pyrogens*. It is not known whether the activators of fever induce the production of an endogenous pyrogenlike protein.

c. *Fever and the Central Nervous System*. Clearly, as in other vertebrates, some pyrogenic mediator leads to an elevation in the thermoregulatory set-point and this results in the fishes actively elevating their body temperature.

It is unknown what the final mediator of fever is in fishes. It is known, however, that the drug acetaminophen, a commonly used antipyretic drug for mammals, does result in attentuation of fever in fishes (Reynolds 1977).

Summary

Five of the seven extant classes of vertebrates have been tested for their febrile responses. All five classes have been shown to have representatives which develop fever in response to some common activators such as Gram-negative bacteria. Figure 41 summarizes much of our current understanding of the comparative biology of fever. On the basis of the many similarities in the febrile responses among the vertebrates, it appears likely that fever is a primitive trait having a long phylogenetic history. It is probable that primitive bony fishes, some 400 millions years ago, were responding to bacterial infection by developing a fever.

It is unknown whether representatives of the classes Agnatha (lampreys, etc.) and Chondrichthyes (sharks, etc.) develop fevers. A fascinating article by Casterlin and Reynolds (1977b) has shown that the crayfish (*Cambarus bartoni*), an invertebrate belonging to the phylum Arthropoda, also develops a fever following infection with bacteria. Very possibly other species of invertebrates also develop fevers in response to the appropriate activating agent. For example, it would hardly be surprising, at this point, if one found that insects (both ectothermic and endothermic species) developed fevers. The ability of an organism to raise its thermoregulatory set-point in response to some infectious agent might turn out to be a fundamental characteristic of almost all organisms capable of regulating their body temperature.

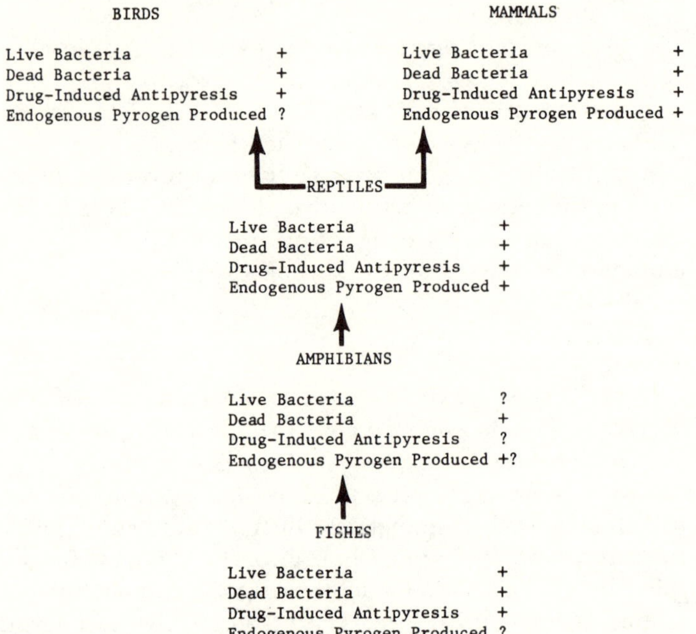

Figure 41. Febrile responses of various vertebrates to injection with live bacteria, dead bacteria (containing the endotoxins), and to dead bacteria along with either sodium salicylate or acetaminophen. Also noted is whether an endogenous pyrogen has been produced by the host's white blood cells. + = positive response; ? = response not yet determined.

4. The Adaptive Value of Fever

Introduction

The role of fever in disease has been debated for literally thousands of years. Reviews concerned with the biology of fever often have ended by raising the question of whether fever is beneficial (see, for example, Dubois 1948; Atkins and Bodel 1972). In 1960, Bennett and Nicastri reviewed this question and, on the basis of the information available to them, were unable to conclude whether fever was a host defense mechanism. Since 1972, however, research into several new areas related to the biology of fever has provided fresh insight into this question. This last chapter will review the literature, past and present, which is pertinent to an understanding of the function of fever. As the bulk of the evidence now seems to support the thesis that fever has an adaptive function, this chapter will also include a section on the possible mechanisms behind fever's beneficial role.

Historical Observations

A. Hippocrates to Liebermeister

Hippocrates (460-357 B.C.E.) had great faith in the healing power of nature ("Nature never needs any instruction") (Major 1954). Much of Hippocrates' philosophy of medicine was rooted in the doctrine of humors. This doctrine was based largely on the notion of Empedocles (490-430 B.C.E.) that the human body was composed of the four elements of earth, air, fire, and water. These concepts were expanded by others, most notably Hippocrates, to correspond to the four "humors" of the body: blood, phlegm, yellow bile, and black bile. According to Yost (1950), the humoral theory of disease maintained that illness was caused when one of the four bodily humors was produced excessively. Once this happened, the body's defenses came into action as demonstrated by the patient's raised body temperature (fever). The excess humor was thus "cooked," separated, and eventually evacuated. As a result, it is not surprising that Hippocrates believed that fever was a beneficial symptom during disease. For example, in one of his writings, he stated that during an ulcerative eye infection "a fever supervening is favourable" (Coxe 1846).

Rufus of Ephesus (ca. 100 A.C.E.) was another famous physician who strongly believed that fever had a beneficial effect. He wrote, "I think that you cannot find another drug which heats in a more penetrating manner than fever; for this reason it is a good remedy for an individual seized with convulsions, and if there were a physician skillful enough to produce a fever, it would be useless to seek any other remedy against disease" (Major 1954). Rufus advocated the use of fever as a therapeutic agent in various disease states including epilepsy, convulsions, tetany, asthma, melancholia, and certain skin diseases. It is thought that the fevers Rufus advocated using to cure these diseases were malarial in origin. This concept of "fever therapy" reappeared many centuries later and will be discussed in detail in the next section of this chapter.

The effects of these early physicians on Western man's thoughts concerning fever and disease persisted through the eighteenth century. For example, the belief that fever was beneficial received no greater support than from Thomas Sydenham (1624-1689), the noted English physician. Sydenham, apparently influenced by the writings of Hippocrates, wrote that "fever is Nature's engine which she brings into the field to remove her enemy" (Payne 1900).

By Liebermeister's time this view of fever was changing (Liebermeister 1887). Recall that Liebermeister was the physician who extensively studied the biology of fever and was the first to accurately define "fever" as the regulation of body temperature at a higher level. While not denying fever's adaptive function, Liebermeister believed that fevers were dangerous if they were too high or persisted for too long. He hypothesized that the positive aspects of fever were related to the effects of high temperatures on the growth of microorganisms. The dangers of fever were thought to be related to a general body wasting leading to a reduction in body weight, appetite, and a degeneration of organs. Nevertheless, Liebermeister urged that antipyretic drug therapy be used only for high fevers of long duration ("cutting off the peaks"). He thought that fevers of moderate magnitude, or those of high magnitude (if they occurred for a short period of time) were actually beneficial.

Based on the often indiscriminate utilization of antipyretic drugs to reduce all fevers in modern times, it would appear that contrary to historical beliefs, it is now generally thought that fever is harmful. One might surmise from this widespread attempt to reduce fevers that convincing evidence had been presented which demonstrated that fevers were harmful. This is not the case. If anything, the weight of evidence tends to support the opposite conclusion. Why then have antipyretic drugs been so widely prescribed? Perhaps the answer to this question is related to the other effects of such antipyretic drugs as the salicylates and indomethacin. Not only do these drugs reduce fever, but at the same time they are also analgesics (reduce pain). It is possible that a drug which is purely antipyretic would have no effect on the pain which accompanies most infections. But these drugs, by having a dual function, may lead the individual to believe that his feeling better is a direct result of the lowering of his fever.

One aspect of fever which has received a great deal of attention is fever therapy. This actually is not directly relevant to the question of the role of naturally occurring fever. In fever therapy the body temperature of the individual is raised above that which is normally encountered in response to the infecting agent. However, since in almost every discussion of fever's function, the role of fever therapy comes up, it is worthwhile to review this phenomenon briefly. Furthermore, a discussion of fever therapy does help to better define the possible mechanisms by which the elevation of body temperature may or may not be helpful.

B. Fever Therapy

Ever since Hippocrates' time, it had been observed that the rare cases of cure or of long-lasting remissions of "progressive paralysis" were often preceded by an infectious disease accompanied by a high fever. By 1858 Esmarck and Jessen had established the link between "progressive paralysis" and syphilis (Wagner-Jauregg 1927). Although apparently unaware of Rufus' suggestions concerning malarial fevers as a form of therapy some 1,800 years earlier, Wagner-Jauregg in 1887 proposed that the inoculation of malaria might be a justifiable means of treating cases of general paralysis or neurosyphilis (Wagner-Jauregg 1927). The rationale behind the use of malarial pathogens to induce a fever was that malaria could be effectively treated with quinine, thereby exchanging an incurable disease (syphilis) for one that could be more easily managed or controlled (malaria). Further support for the potential therapeutic value of malaria-induced fevers was provided by the knowledge that in certain areas of the world, such as India and China, where both syphilis and malaria were endemic, cases of neurosyphilis were rare (Solomon et al. 1926).

It was not until 1917 that Wagner-Jauregg tested this hypothesis. Nine persons suffering from paralysis attributable to syphilis were injected with the infectious blood of malarial patients. In three of the nine patients, recovery from paralysis was practically complete (Wernstedt 1927). This led to further experimentation and clinical observations in literally thousands of patients. Before the malarial treatment, only 1% of patients showed full remission from "progressive paralysis." Wagner-Jauregg's fever therapy led to remissions in over 30%, based on a sample size in the thousands. For his work on fever therapy, Wagner-Jauregg was awarded the Nobel Prize in Physiology and Medicine in 1927.

Other forms of venereal disease were also treated with fever therapy. For example, typhoid vaccine was used for resistant forms of gonorrhea. Providing fevers were above 40°C, these treatments were moderately successful (Knight et al. 1943). There were, however, some severe side effects to these treatments. For example, not only did these Gram-negative bacteria induce a fever, but these agents occasionally resulted in severe hypotension or cardiovascular shock.

The mechanisms behind the successful treatment of neurosyphilis and other forms of venereal disease by fever inducing agents are thought to be related to one or more of three general effects.

1. The first is the direct effect of high temperature on the pathogenic organism. It is possible that the pathogens responsible for venereal disease or other diseases might not grow or even survive at the elevated or febrile temperatures. As an example, it is known that the gonococcus responsible for gonorrhea is killed outright at temperatures of 40°C (Speirer 1931).

2. The second possible mechanism is more indirect, but still relates to the elevation in body temperature induced by the pyrogens. It is possible that an elevated body temperature leads to an increase in host defense mechanisms (e.g. possibly increasing antibody production, leukocyte phagocytosis, etc.). The direct and indirect effects of high temperature on pathogenic organisms will be discussed in more detail later in this chapter.

3. The third possible mechanism behind the successful treatment of diseases using pyrogens could be related to the action of these activating agents on some other aspects of the immune system. For example, it is known that typhoid or typhoid-paratyphoid vaccine leads to an improvement in a variety of eye and related ailments (Bennett and Cluff 1957; Ellis and Smith 1973). The use of these fever-inducing agents, however, is thought to be related to the effects of the endotoxins of these Gram-negative bacteria on the adrenal glands, resulting in an increased secretion of the anti-inflammatory hormone, cortisol, and not to an elevation in body temperature.

Another area in which fever therapy has had a moderate amount of success has been as an antitumor agent (Cavaliere et al. 1967; Suit and Schwayder 1974; Overgaard 1977). For more than a hundred years, a link between high temperatures and tumor regressions has been noted in the medical literature (Cavaliere et al. 1967). In 1893, a New York physician, William Coley, began to treat various forms of cancer by infecting individuals with "Coley's toxins," living cultures of *Streptococcus sp*. often mixed with other species of bacteria (Nauts et al. 1953). Coley apparently had some success with this form of cancer therapy. It is not apparent from the literature whether the regression of these tumors was related to the induced fevers or to some other effect of the bacteria on the immune responses of the diseased individual.

It is known, however, that high temperatures do have an adverse effect on many types of tumor cells (Cavaliere et al. 1967; Suzuki 1967; Love et al. 1970; Suit and Schwayder 1974; Overgaard 1977). In a recent review on the effects of high temperatures on malignant cells, Overgaard (1977) has concluded that various types of malignant cells, when heated to between 41° and 43°C, appear to be selectively destroyed by the heat. The mechanisms behind the adverse effects of temperature on tumor cells have been broken down into several categories. The first is related to the effects of high temperatures on RNA, DNA, and protein synthesis. High temperatures result in an inhibition of cellular activities related to RNA and DNA. These adverse effects are not, however, restricted to tumor cells. Another effect of high temperatures appears to be that of markedly depressing various metabolic or cellular respiratory processes of tumor cells. This effect appears to be primarily restricted to tumor, and not to healthy, cells. A third effect of heat is that of increasing the development of lysosomes in the cytoplasm of tumor cells. Lysosomes are intracellular particles which contain large amounts of degradative enzymes. As such, the presence of increased amounts of these enzymes might suggest increased tumor cell destruction. In fact, there is evidence of increased lysosomal enzyme activity after heat treatment. Apparently tumor cell lysosomes, in contrast to nonmalignant cells, not only increase their numbers but also tend to be more sensitive to heat, thereby releasing more of their degradative enzymes.

Overgaard summarizes the effects of heat on malignant

tumors by concluding that the use of hyperthermia in conjunction with other forms of treatment such as irradiation and chemotherapy might, under certain circumstances, reduce the doses of highly toxic chemotherapeutic agents which must currently be used in clinical practice.

Fever and Survival—Studies Involving Mammals

Studies which have specifically related to the question of fever's function can be conveniently divided into three general categories—correlation, antipyresis, and hyper-hypothermia studies. In correlation studies, the magnitude of the febrile response of some organism to an infectious agent is compared to some aspect of the host's immunological defense mechanisms. The simplest comparison is between fever and mortality rate. As in all correlative studes, it is impossible to determine whether the correlated variables have a casual relationship (e.g. does smoking cause lung cancer) or only an association (e.g. people with the likelihood of developing lung cancer also have the tendency to smoke). The second type of study involves the use of antipyretic agents to reduce the fever of an organism (lower its set-point) and then, as in the correlation studies, the magnitude of the fever is compared with some aspect of the host's physiological state such as mortality or morbidity rate. The problem with these studies is that in the process of producing antipyresis, drugs are generally used which produce many side effects, some undoubtedly helpful and others harmful. As such, the results of these studies are difficult to interpret. The third type of study involves the use of high or low environmental temperatures to alter the body temperature of infected organisms. These types of studies do not actually affect the fever of the organism since they do not alter its set-point; rather, they only affect its body temperature. These infected organism will be either hypo- or hyperthermic and will be attempting to raise or lower their body temperature to achieve an equilibrium between their core temperature and their set-point temperature. Since hypo- and hyperthermia lead to an increase in various autonomic reflexes which are not found in animals that are normothermic, the results of these investigations are also difficult to interpret. With this brief introduction into the hazards of interpreting data obtained from investigations into the role of fever in disease, the results of these three types of experiments are described below.

A. Correlation Studies

Clinical studies involving human beings generally have shown that the magnitude of the fever is associated with the severity of the infection (Bennett and Nicastri 1960). As a result, patients with the highest fevers tend to have the highest mortality rate. The difficulty with studies involving human beings is that they are completely uncontrolled. Often the results are confounded because some patients receive certain drugs which others do not receive. Furthermore, the patients clearly have not been infected with identical doses of pathogens. To properly perform (from a scientific standpoint) survival studies on human beings, one must infect subjects with identical doses of pathogens, administer no drugs, and then compare their resultant fevers with their mortality or morbidity rates. Clearly, these experiments would be totally unethical. However, what we now have are simply clinical impressions and as such it is impossible to determine from these types of studies whether fever has a beneficial role.

In 1975, Vaughn and Kluger initiated a series of experiments to determine whether there was a correlation between the magnitude of the fever during bacterial infection and the survival rate of laboratory rabbits. These studies used male New Zealand white rabbits which were all about the same age and which came from the same animal supplier. The body temperature of each rabbit was continuously recorded via a thermocouple implanted into its abdomen. These rabbits were injected with two doses of live *Pasteurella multocida*, a Gram-negative bacterium pathogenic to rabbits. In order to prevent possible diurnal variations in survival rate and temperature response, injections of the bacteria were made at approximately the same time of day in each experiment.

The mortality rate of the rabbits was monitored over a five-day period, and all rabbits which were alive at the end of this time were considered survivors. To determine a rabbit's fever, its average temperature over the twenty-four-hour period beginning six hours after injection of bacteria was compared to its average temperature on the control day. This twenty-four-hour period was used because most of the mortality (76% of those rabbits injected with the high dose of bacteria) occurred within this period. The first six hours were excluded since the animals were just in the process of becoming severely ill during this time period. The fevers were than correlated with survival rate. The rabbits were grouped into fever ranges of 0.75°C. These fever ranges were chosen because they were small enough to show clearly the relationship between fever and survival. Smaller fever ranges could not be used for statistical purposes since there were too few animals in each range.

The average abdominal temperature during the control period and after injection of the high dose of bacteria is shown in Figure 42. The mean control day temperature, calculated by averaging the twenty-four hours before injection, was 39.6° ± 0.3°C. The average temperature during the

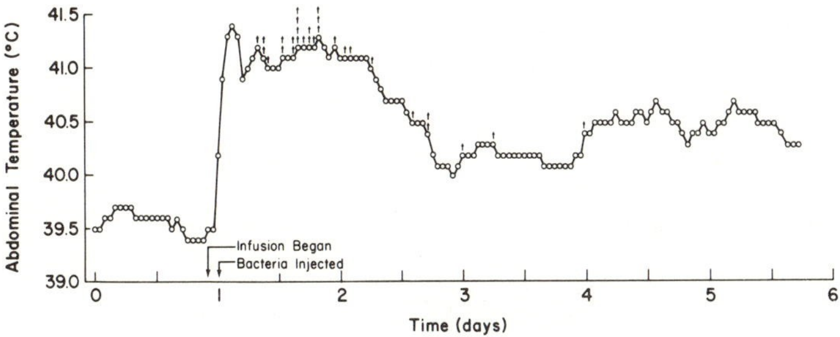

Figure 42. Average abdominal temperature of forty-six rabbits infused with saline and infected with *P. multocida*. Crosses indicate the death of a rabbit.

twenty-four-hour period beginning six hours after injection of bacteria was 41.1° ± 0.7°C.

The correlation between the magnitude of fever developed by the rabbits infected with the high dose of bacteria and the survival rate is shown in Figure 43. Most rabbits developed a fever of less than 2.25°C, and within this temperature range, there is an increase in survival rate as body temperature is elevated. A small number of animals (n = 6) developed fevers above 2.25°C, and showed a decrease in survival rate. The difference in survival rate between animals with less than 1.5 degrees fever and those with greater than 1.5 degrees fever is statistically significant (P <0.02,

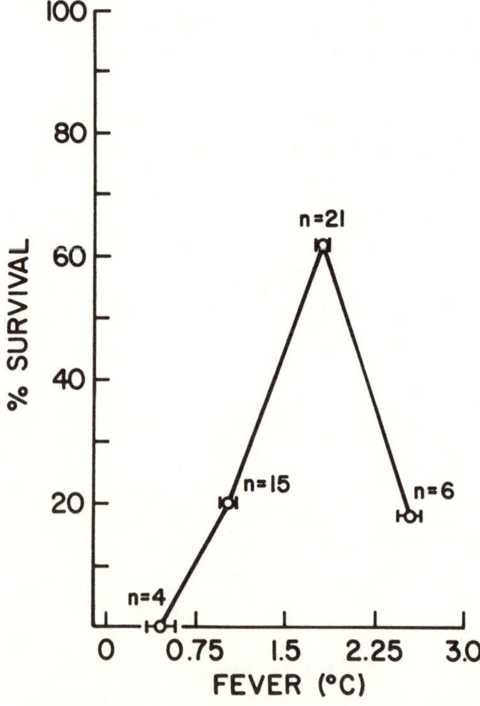

Figure 43. Correlation between the magnitude of fever and the percent survival of forty-six rabbits infected with *P. multocida*. The difference in survival between rabbits with less than 1.5°C fevers and those with greater than 1.5°C fevers is statistically significant.

Chi-squared test) (Vaughn and Kluger 1977; Kluger and Vaughn, 1978).

Another correlation study has recently been reported by Toms et al. (1977). In this study, ferrets (*Mustela sp.*) were infected with different strains of influenza viruses and the resultant fever was correlated with the presence of live viruses in their nasal passages. Groups of three to six nonimmune ferrets were inoculated intranasally with a constant dose of virus. At four-hour intervals, the nasal passages were washed and the fluid was collected and assayed for the presence of live virus. Statistically significant ($P < 0.01$) negative correlations were found between the ferrets' rectal temperatures and the presence of live viruses in the nasal washes, suggesting that fever might lead to the inactivation of viruses.

Clearly, the results of correlation studies involving fever and mortality (Vaughn and Kluger 1977) or fever and morbidity (Toms et al. 1977) are consistent with the theory that fever has a beneficial function.

B. Antipyretic Studies

There have been few studies in which a population of mammals has been infected with identical amounts of pathogens and the effects of antipyresis on mortality or morbidity quantified. One such study, by Klastersky (1971), involved rabbits which were injected with pneumococcal bacteria and then treated with various drugs. Some rabbits were treated with the antipyretic and anti-inflammatory steroid, cortisol. (For some reason, all of these rabbits were also treated with penicillin.) The fever index which developed in the control rabbits (those receiving bacteria + penicillin) was about 3 ½ times that of the experimental rabbits (those receiving bacteria + penicillin + cortisol). The mortality rates were 66% for the control population and 46% for the experimental population. While the mortality rate for the experimental population was reduced, these rabbits did have a greater persistence of pneumococcus. Klastersky suggested that it was the suppression of fever that led to the decreased mortality rate in these rabbits.

These results led Klastersky to attempt to do a double-blind study using human beings in which betamethasone, a potent anti-inflammatory steroid, was administered to patients suffering from severe bacterial infections. As in the above study on rabbits, antibiotic drugs were administered. Again, as in rabbits, the patients receiving the steroids had considerably reduced fevers compared to controls receiving placebos. Klastersky found, however, that not only did the use of these drugs lead to no benefit, but "on the contrary, the infection was more difficult to eradicate in corticoid-treated patients."

These experiments of Klastersky's are particularly difficult to interpret. One aspect of his study which makes interpretation impossible is that all subjects (rabbits or people) received antibiotic drugs. If one is specifically interested in the effects of fever on mortality rate, then from a scientific standpoint, the use of antibiotic drugs should be excluded. The second difficulty with his experiments involves his choice of antipyretic drugs—various types of corticosteroids. While these drugs have some antipyretic activity, they are best known for their powerful effects on the immune response. These steroids suppress inflammation and are used to treat various allergic diseases, asthma, eye and skin diseases, intestinal irritations, etc. (Haynes and Larner 1975). As a result of their potent immuno-suppressive effects, the corticosteroids are seldom prescribed as antipyretic agents. Therefore, one cannot determine if the decrease in mortality in the rabbits treated with cortisol was related to the antipyretic or anti-inflammatory effect of these drugs.

Vaughn and Kluger (1977) have investigated the effects of antipyretic drug therapy on the survival of bacterially infected rabbits. As in their study described above, rabbits were infected with live *P. multocida* and their mortality rate was monitored for a five-day period. In these experiments, half the rabbits received, in addition to the injection of live bacteria, a continuous infusion of antipyretic drugs (100 ml/day of 3 mg/ml sodium salicylate and 10 mg/ml acetaminophen dissolved in sterile, pyrogen-free, saline). A combination of antipyretic drugs was used because it was found that either drug, by itself, produced no antipyresis. Control rabbits received the injection of live bacteria plus a continuous infusion of sterile, pyrogen-free, saline (100 ml/day). As in their correlation study, the rabbit's twenty-four-hour fevers were grouped into fever ranges of 0.75°C.

Even with these high doses of antipyretic drugs, very little antipyresis was induced. For example, when the high dose of bacteria was administered, the average decrease in body temperature of the antipyretic-treated rabbits, compared to the saline-treated rabbits, was only 0.32°C. While this difference was small, it was, nevertheless, highly statistically significant ($P < 0.005$).

A comparison of the survival rate between bacterially infected rabbits infused with saline and those infused with antipyretic drugs is shown in Figure 44. The curve relating fever to the percent survival was shifted upward and to the left in the antipyretic-treated rabbits. Now there were no longer any rabbits with average fevers greater than 2.25°C, and therefore the percent survival increased. On the other hand, more rabbits were now in the low fever range of 0° to 0.75°C average fever (11 vs. 4) where more animals died. However, in any fever range (0°-0.75°, 0.75°-1.50°, or 1.50°-225°C) the percent survival of the rabbits receiving antipyretic drugs was *increased*. Overall, the percent survival of the saline controls was 37% and that of the antipyretic-treated rabbits was 51%. This difference was statistically significant ($P < 0.05$).

It is likely, therefore, that some side effect of sodium salicylate or acetaminophen, *not related to their effect on body temperature*, influenced the survival of bacterially infected rabbits. For example, aspirin is known to inhibit the vascular reactivity to substances released in response to endotoxins (catecholamines, histamine, seratonin, bradykinin) and to inhibit edema (Woodbury and Fingle 1975). Furthermore, pretreatment of various laboratory animals with antipyretic drugs such as acetylsalicylic acid or indomethacin has been shown to antagonize the vasodepressive actions of endo-

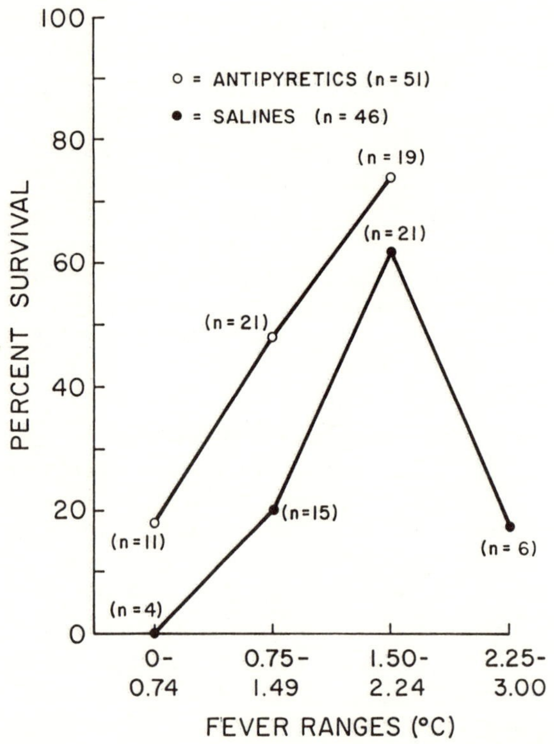

Figure 44. Correlation between the magnitude of fever and the percent survival of rabbits infected with *P. multocida* and infused with either saline or antipyretic drugs. Note that none of the rabbits receiving antipyretic drugs developed fevers in the 2.25°-3.00°C range. On the other hand, there are now more rabbits receiving antipyretic drugs in the low fever range of 0°-0.74°C, compared to the saline controls. Overall, however, the use of these drugs led to an increase in the percent survival of the rabbits. This increase was not related to the effects of these drugs on the body temperatures of these rabbits, and remains unexplained.

toxins, thus diminishing the likelihood of cardiovascular shock, or the severe lowering of blood pressure (Greenway and Murthy 1971; Parratt and Sturgess 1974).

Based on these known anti-inflammatory effects of sodium salicylate and, to a lesser extent, acetaminophen, we speculated that the drug-treated rabbits would have a diminished inflammatory response and might therefore be less likely to become hypotensive. We hypothesized that the mean arterial pressure of the infected saline controls would therefore be lower than in those receiving the anti-inflammatory drugs, and that this difference in mean arterial pressure might partially account for the difference in mortality. To test this hypothesis, rabbits were implanted with a catheter in their carotid artery and their mean arterial pressure was monitored for several days. During a twenty-four-hour control period, the mean arterial pressure of loosely restrained, unanesthetized rabbits was about 87 mm Hg. Following the injection of live bacteria, the mean arterial pressure fell by about 15 mm Hg in both groups (saline-control and drug-treated rabbits). Blood pressure remained depressed for over forty hours. Since most mortality occurred within the first twenty-four hours, these data were interpreted to indicate that the increase in survival of the drug-treated rabbits is not related to any effect of these drugs on their mean arterial pressure (Malvin et al. 1978). It is not currently known why the animals receiving the drug therapy had a lower mortality rate.

As in the case of Klastersky's experiments, ours are difficult to interpret. Clearly these "antipyretic" drugs have other effects besides that of lowering body temperature. The data presented in Figure 44 are, however, consistent with the hypothesis that low fevers and high fevers are harmful and that the optimal fever to develop during a bacterial infection is about 2°C. Antipyresis of high fevers to more moderate levels is beneficial; antipyresis of moderate fevers to very low fevers is harmful. It must be strongly emphasized that none of these experiments has, in any way, conclusively resolved the question of fever's function.

C. Hyperthermia and Hypothermia Studies

Kass and his associates have injected endotoxins into mice and rats and have found that raising the environmental temperature resulted in an "artificial fever" which increased the susceptibility of these animals to the lethal action of endotoxin (Connor and Kass 1961; Porter and Kass 1962). Atwood and Kass (1964) found that when rabbits were placed at a high environmental temperature of 37°C, their body temperature was elevated by about 2°C. Following injection with endotoxins, these hyperthermic rabbits still developed fevers, although the magnitudes of these fevers were not as great as those in rabbits maintained at a room temperature of 23°C. The rabbits which were hyperthermic had as much as a sixtyfold increase in their sensitivity to the lethal effects of these endotoxins. When rabbits were shorn of their fur, they invariably responded to endotoxic challenge at room temperature by becoming hypothermic. These rabbits were resistant to the lethal action of endotoxins (Atwood and Kass 1964). They concluded that the "induction of fever increases the lethal action of endotoxin and conversely, the prevention of fever exerts a protective effect against such a lethal challenge."

There is an obvious difficulty in attempting to apply the results of the above studies to resolving whether fever is adaptive or maladaptive during disease. Clearly, the effects of injections of endotoxins are considerably different from those which occur during infection with live bacteria, or viruses. For example, it is known that injection of lethal doses of endotoxin leads to an acute fall in arterial blood pressure (Greenway and Murthy 1971). It is generally assumed that it is this "endotoxic shock" which is the immediate cause of death in response to large doses of endotoxin. Inducing hyperthermia in an animal would undoubtedly lead to an increased sensitivity to the hypotensive effects of large doses of endotoxins for at least two reasons. First, the hyperthermic animal would be peripherally vasodilated. This would result in an effective decrease in the central blood volume and would lead to reflexes which would increase heart rate and stroke volume in order for the animal to maintain its blood pressure at normal levels. The second effect of hyperthermia would be that, whether via the respiratory tract, via the skin, or elsewhere, the hyperthermic organism would lose greater amounts of water by evaporation. This reduction in total body water would further compromise blood volume and make the maintenance of a normal blood pressure difficult. Therefore, in response to any further stress, such as the effects of endotoxins on vascular permeability, it seems reasonable that these heat stressed animals would be particularly sensitive. Clearly, the effects of body temperature on endotoxin-induced mortality could have little to do directly with the effects of fever on mortality due to infectious agents.

Klastersky (1971) also performed survival studies on rabbits which were made hypothermic by shaving their fur. Recall that Klastersky injected these rabbits with pneumococcal bacteria and then treated all of them with penicillin. Those rabbits which were shaved developed considerably lower fevers than did the control rabbits. The mortality rate of the control rabbits was 46% and that of the shaved rabbits only 31%. Again, as in his experiments involving the administration of cortisol, the suppression of fever favored the persistence of the bacteria. For example, after eighteen hours had elapsed, the blood of 100% of the control rabbits was sterile but the blood of only 80% of the hypothermic (shaved) rabbits was sterile. These data would suggest that a fever in response to pneumococcal infection in the laboratory rabbit increased the mortality rate but decreased the morbidity rate. However, as described above, all the rabbits received the antibiotic drug penicillin, thus making interpretation difficult.

Many other studies which have involved the induction of hypo- or hyperthermia in pneumococcal-infected animals have led to essentially the opposite results of those reported by Klastersky. For example, in 1909, Strouse demonstrated that the natural resistance pigeons had to pneumococci was related to their normal body temperature of about 41.5°C. When their body temperatures were reduced by ice or by the administration of drugs, they became susceptible to the infection and died. Similar findings were reported by Muschenheim et al. (1943) for pneumococcal infections in rabbits. These animals were infected with pneumococci, and hypothermia was induced by one of several methods so that the rectal temperatures of these rabbits were maintained between 30° and 34°C. Control rabbits were infected and had their body temperature maintained at normal to low febrile levels, between 39° and 41°C. All of the hypothermic rabbits died, whereas only five of the thirty-one control rabbits died. These authors concluded that hypothermia was clearly harmful to the infected host and that the development of fever led to an enhancement of the host defense mechanism.

An area which has recently begun to receive attention is that of the febrile responses of newborns. It has been known for a long time that many newborn mammals had a fairly labile body temperature during their first few days of life (Pembrey 1895). Furthermore, in response to infection, newborn human infants (Haahr and Mogensen 1977) or other infant mammals such as rabbits (Satinoff et al. 1976) tend to have a limited febrile response. Satinoff et al. have shown, however, that newborn rabbits, while not raising their body temperature by physiological means following an injection of endotoxin, will raise their body temperature by behavioral means. When injected with *Pseudomonas* endotoxins and allowed to select a range of environmental temperatures, these rabbits selected a warmer environmental temperature, resulting in an elevation in their body temperatures. These results were similar to those reported following injections of endotoxins in ectothermic vertebrates such as lizards, frogs, and fishes.

Haahr and Mogensen (1977) believe that hyperthermia (or more precisely a rise in body temperature) during certain viral infections is beneficial to newborns. To support their claim, they cite several studies which have demonstrated that elevations in body temperature during various viral infections have reduced the mortality rate in newborn mice, dogs, and human beings. For example, Teisner and Haahr (1974) found that when two-to-three-day-old mice were infected with Coxsackie virus and held at an environmental temperature of 34°C, they had a mean body temperature of 35.8°C, some 2° to 3°C higher than control mice held at room temperature of 22° to 24°C. Those mice which were held at 34°C had a considerably lower mortality rate than did the control mice. Carmichael et al. (1969) reported similar findings for two-to-five-day-old dog pups which were inoculated with canine herpesvirus. When the pups were held at an environmental temperature of 28° to 30°C, they had a rectal temperature of about 35° to 37°C; those held at an environmental temperature of 36.7 to 37.7°C had a rectal temperature of 38.3° to 39.4°C, approximately normal rectal temperatures for adult dogs. Following inoculation with herpesvirus, those dogs with the lower rectal temperatures all died within eight days, whereas those with the higher rectal temperatures all survived nine days or longer. The authors of this study concluded that the elevation of the body temperature to the adult level was beneficial to the infected pups. Based on these data, Haahr and Mogensen (1977) suggest that one of the reasons that generalized herpes-simplex infections are greatly overrepresented in premature babies might be attributable to their restricted temperature regulation and poor febrile response.

The entire subject of the effects of hyperthermia and hypothermia on the course of infection through the year 1960 is discussed in greater detail in Bennett and Nicastri's excellent review (1960). While it is difficult to draw definitive conclusions concerning the role of fever in disease based on hyper- or hypothermia studies, the weight of the evidence supports an adaptive function for fever during infections with certain bacterial or viral pathogens.

Fever and Survival—Studies Involving Nonmammalian Vertebrates

The use of the comparative method has been a potent tool in the hands of experimental biologists and has allowed them to select the most appropriate animal model to answer their specific questions. The renowned scientist A. V. Hill summarized the elegance of this approach as follows: "By the methods of comparative physiology or of experimental biology, by the choice of a suitable organ, tissue or process, in some animal far removed in evolution we may often throw light upon some function or process in the higher animals or man" (Ratliff 1967).

Great care must be taken in selecting an experimental animal. It is important that the species selected for investigation be able to provide results that can be extrapolated to the organism in which the investigator is specifically interested. Generally, the more stable the characteristic which is being studied, the more readily one can extrapolate from the results obtained from a "lower" vertebrate to a "higher" vertebrate such as man. Fever, as we have seen in Chapter 3, is particularly conservative throughout the vertebrates, with species from fishes through mammals developing fevers in response to inoculation with the appropriate activators. Other characteristics of the febrile response, such as the production of endogenous pyrogens, and the effects of antipyretic drugs, also support the hypothesis that fever has been a component of the immune response of vertebrates for over 400 million years. In endotherms such as birds and mammals, the maintenance of a body temperature of 2° or 3°C above afebrile levels often results in an increase in their energy consumption by 20% or more. This is the result of the Q_{10} effect of increased temperature on various biochemical reactions. In the ectothermic vertebrates the amount of excess energy expended during a fever is unknown. However, since this requires considerable movement by the febrile organism, it undoubtedly leads to increased energy expenditure. Furthermore, as in the endothermic vertebrates, the maintenance of an elevated body temperature will likely also result in an approximately 20% increase in energy consumption. If fever did not have an adaptive function, then it woud be unlikely that this energetically expensive phenomenon would have persisted for millions of years in at least six orders of mammals and invertebrate classes from the bony fishes through the birds.

In addition to the above "economic" argument for a beneficial role for fever in the vertebrates, there have appeared several studies specifically involving the role of fever in disease in reptiles and fishes. The results of these investigations are described below.

A. Fever and Survival in Reptiles

The advantage of using an ectotherm to investigate the role of fever in disease is that following injection with some pathogenic organism, the rise in body temperature can be prevented simply by preventing the ectotherm from moving to a warmer microclimate.

Recall that the lizard, *D. dorsalis*, when placed in a chamber which has a temperature range, will select a preferred environmental temperature resulting in a mean body temperature of about 38°C. Furthermore, following inoculation with Gram-negative bacteria, these lizards select a warmer environmental temperature resulting in a fever of 2° to 4°C. To investigate whether this rise in body temperature has any survival value, lizards were injected with live *A. hydrophila* and placed in incubators at 34°, 36°, 38°, 40°, and 42°C (Kluger et al. 1975). Control lizards were inoculated with saline and then placed into the incubators. The results of this study are shown in Figure 45.

The relation between the lizards' temperatures and percentage survival following bacterial infection was highly significant ($P < 0.005$). Within twenty-four hours, approximately 50% of the lizards maintained at 38°C were dead. However, lizards maintained at 40° and 42°C had only 14% and 0% mortality, respectively. Conversely, lizards maintained at 36° and 34°C experienced mortalities of 66% and 75%, respectively. After three and a half days, all the lizards at 34°C were dead. After seven days the percentage mortalities were: 42°C, 25%; 40°C, 33%; 38°C and 36°C, 75%; and 34°C, 100%. In contrast, lizards injected with saline and maintained at 34°, 38°, and 42°C for seven days experienced 0%, 0%, and 34% mortality, respectively.

At the highest temperature tested, the pattern of deaths was similar for the controls and the infected lizards. Whereas most deaths occurred within three and a half days in infected lizards maintained at 34° to 40°C, virtually all deaths at 42°C occurred after three and a half days. Apparently, maintenance at 42°C for a period exceeding three and a half days is harmful in itself. This suggests that the deaths

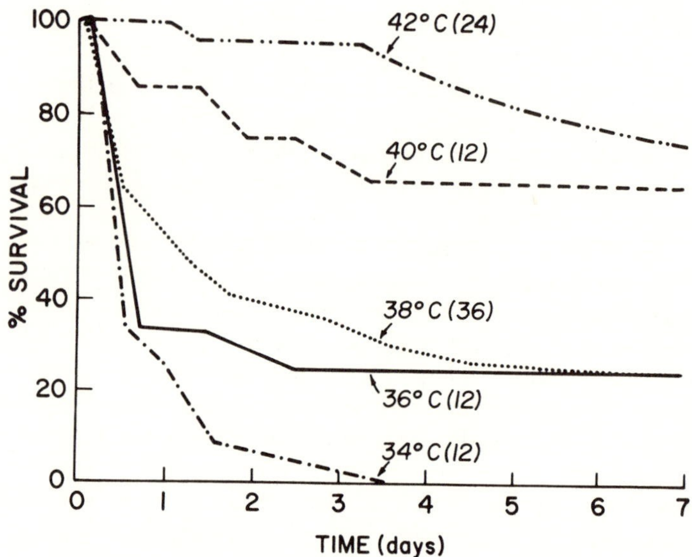

Figure 45. Percentage survival of desert iguanas infected with *A. hydrophila* and maintained at temperatures of 34° to 42°C. The number of lizards in each group is given in parenthesis. (From Kluger et al. 1975.)

at 42°C were not due to the bacterial infection, but to some undetermined adverse effect of long-term elevation in body temperature.

These results supported the hypothesis that fever following a bacterial infection was beneficial to the host. This received further support in a subsequent study by Bernheim and Kluger (1976b). In this study, the lizards were also infected with live *A. hydrophila*, but now they were allowed to select their preferred body temperature in the simulated desert environment (see Figure 37).

The lizards infected with the live bacteria developed a daytime fever averaging 2.3°C over a five-day period (mean body temperature was 40.6°C). Because the heat lamps were off at night, the lizards could thermoregulate only during the daylight hours. By day 6, body temperatures had returned to the afebrile levels. One of these thirteen lizards did not develop a fever and died on day 3, while one lizard that did develop a fever died on day 7. (We defined a fever as an increase in body temperature of 0.6°C or greater, in agreement with the United States Pharmacopeia [1975] definition of fever in rabbits.) Of those lizards that developed a fever, 92% survived the seven-day experiment, a value in agreement with that found in an earlier study (Kluger et al. 1975). These data also demonstrated that an elevation in body temperature need not be continuous since the lizard's body temperatures were lowered at night. Lizards injected with saline alone did not develop any fever, and all survived.

Another part of the experiments by Bernheim and Kluger (1976b) involved the use of the antipyretic drug sodium salicylate to attenuate the fevers in the lizards. In these experiments, twelve lizards were injected with the live bacteria along with a dose of sodium salicylate, which produced antipyresis in seven of the twelve lizards. All five febrile lizards survived, while the seven afebrile lizards died (Figure 46). To determine whether the dose of sodium salicylate used in these experiments was toxic, eight lizards were injected with live bacteria and sodium salicylate and placed inside a constant temperature chamber; their body temperatures were maintained at the febrile level by adjusting the chamber temperature to about 41°C during the day (about the average temperature selected by febrile lizards in the simulated natural environment) and at low temperatures at night (again, as in the simulated natural environment). Only one of these eight lizards died, indicating that the dose of sodium salicylate used in these experiments was not toxic.

These data indicated that the administration of sodium salicylate to these lizards with *A. hydrophila* infections was harmful when it resulted in a reduction in body temperature to the afebrile level. When sodium salicylate failed to produce antipyresis (as in the five lizards in the simulated desert environment or in the eight lizards maintained in the constant temperature chamber), the survival of infected lizards was not adversely affected by the drug. However, before it can be concluded that fever has a general survival function

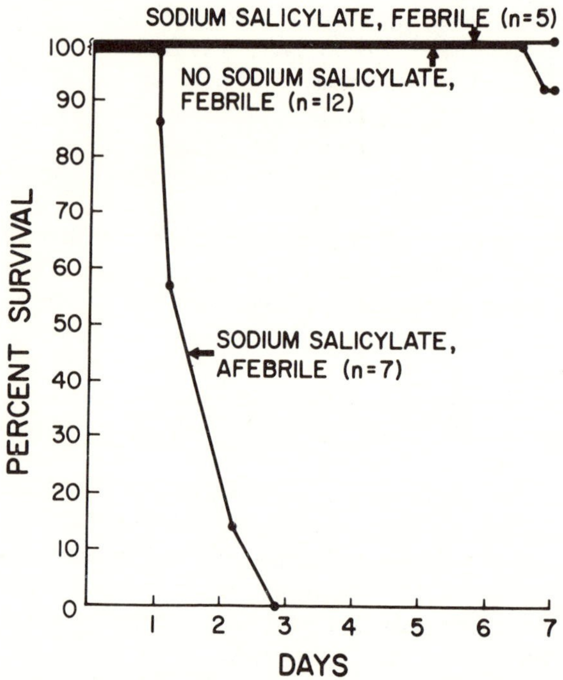

Figure 46. Percentage survival of desert iguanas infected with *A. hydrophila* with and without sodium salicylate. (From Bernheim and Kluger 1976b.)

in reptiles, additional work needs to be done using other pathogenic organisms in these and other species of reptiles.

B. Fever and Survival in Fishes

There have been several studies involving the effects of temperature on the mortality rate of fishes. One of these, by Covert and Reynolds (1977), entailed infecting goldfish with live *A. hydrophila* and monitoring their survival rate over a period of three days. These investigators had previously reported that several species of freshwater fishes developed fevers in response to injections with these bacteria (Reynolds et al. 1976; Reynolds and Covert 1977). In their survival study they infected goldfish and then held them at temperatures of 25.5°, 28.0°, or 30.5°C. These represented, respectively, hypothermic, normothermic, and febrile temperatures. Goldfish maintained at a febrile temperature of 30.5°C had a survival rate of 84%; those maintained at 28.0°C had a survival rate of 64%; those at 25.5°C had a survival rate of 24% (Figure 47). Another ten fish were injected with the same dose of live *A. hydrophila* and were allowed to thermoregulate in a shuttlebox. These fish developed a fever averaging almost 5°C and had a mean body temperature of 32.7°C. None of these fish died. Covert and Reynolds concluded that a fever in response to infection with *A. hydrophila* increases the survival rate of goldfish.

There have been several studies involving the effects of elevations in water (= body) temperature on the mortality rate of various species of freshwater fishes infected with viruses. For example, Watson et al. (1954) reported that sockeye salmon (*Oncorhynchus nerka*) infected with sockeye salmon virus experienced fewer mortalities when held at a water temperature of 20°C than when held at 15.5°C or lower. In 1970, Amend reported similar findings for sockeye salmon infected with hematopoietic necrosis virus

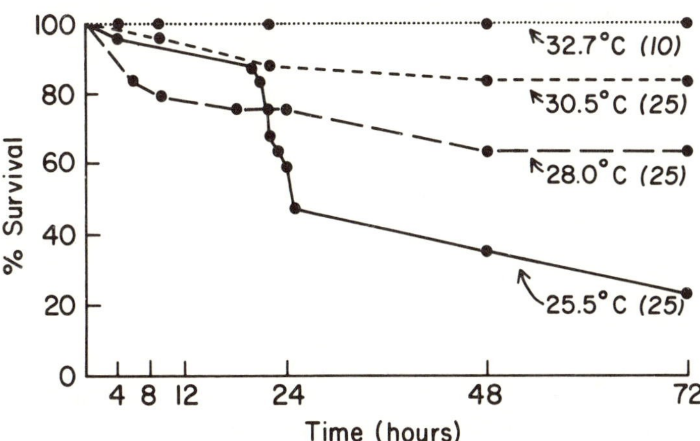

Figure 47. Percent survival of goldfish infected with *A. hydrophila* and maintained at temperatures of 25.5°C, 28.0°C, and 30.5°C; ten goldfish were allowed to behaviorally thermoregulate and selected a mean body temperature of 32.7°C. The number of fish in each group is given in parenthesis. (From Covert and Reynolds 1977.)

(IHN). The mortality rate of salmon held between 12° and 16°C was about 66%, whereas for those held between 18° and 20°C it was only about 30%. Even when there was a delay of up to twenty-four hours before the infected fishes were placed in the warmer environment, there was still a substantial decrease in the mortality rate. Similar results were reported for IHN-infected rainbow trout (*Salmo gairdneri*) (Amend 1976).

One of the difficulties in interpreting the above studies is that since it is unknown whether these fishes develop fevers in response to viral infections, it is unclear whether raising their body temperatures simulates hyperthermia or fever. If the former were the case, then the beneficial effects of raising the body temperatures of these fishes would simply be a form of fever therapy and, therefore, these results would not be applicable to a discussion of the role of fever in disease. Since several species of freshwater fishes develop fevers in response to bacterial infection, I believe that it is likely that, given the opportunity, the species of fishes used in the viral studies would also behaviorally select warmer environmental temperatures. If this turns out to be the case, then these results will support the thesis that fever has an adaptive function in fishes.

C. Implications for Birds and Mammals

The results of the studies of the survival value of fever in ectothermic vertebrates have shown that following an infection, a rise in body temperature results in a decrease in their mortality rate. These data provide further support for the belief that fever in the endotherms is also beneficial since it is unlikely that fever would be adaptive in both fishes and reptiles and would have become maladaptive in birds and mammals. It is also likely that during certain infections a fever might play a neutral or even maladaptive role. This is because the evolution of host-pathogen interactions never ceases. As the host evolves new mechanisms for combatting infection (e.g. antibody production, elevation in body temperature, etc.), the pathogen also evolves new mechanisms for successfully parasitizing the host. There undoubtedly develops a symbiotic relationship between the host and its parasite with, in most cases, a balance being achieved. This balance keeps the host immunologically "primed" or prepared in the event it is exposed to some new pathogen.

If fever does, in most cases, have survival value in the endothermic vertebrates, then the widespread use of antipyretic drugs and other agents (e.g. sponge baths) to reduce the body temperature of febrile patients should be reevaluated. At times the elevated temperature of a patient is harmful. For example, when body temperature is over 40° or 41°C, then clearly there is potential harm from heat-related disorders; however, for fevers of less than 40° or 41°C it might be better for the patient to maintain this febrile temperature, as it is likely to enhance his host defense mechanisms. Some of the possible mechanisms behind the survival value of fever will be discussed in the next section of this chapter.

Mechanisms behind the Survival Value of Fever

A. Direct Effect of Temperature on Pathogenic Microorganisms

All organisms have optimal temperature ranges for growth (see Figures 1-3). During infections, an elevation in body temperature of only a few degrees might result in the movement of the pathogenic microorganisms into a range where their growth is severely inhibited, while at the same time the host organism might still be within its optimal temperature zone. In fact, even if the host organism were temporarily pushed out of its optimal range, as long as this did not result in irreversible side effects, then a fever would still be beneficial.

Lwoff (1959 & 1969) has investigated several aspects of the direct effects of temperature on the growth of viruses. He found, for example, that poliomyelities virus was inhibited by febrile body temperatures. The yield of virus grown in tissue culture at 37°C was 250 times greater than that at 40°C. By performing the appropriate experiments, he was able to determine that the viral particles were not destroyed by the higher temperatures, but rather that their development was being impaired (Lwoff 1959). The specific mechanism behind the direct effect of temperature on the impairment of viral growth is not known for certain but is believed to be related to the inhibitory effect of elevated temperature on viral ribonucleic acid (Lwoff 1969).

Some species of viruses seem to grow better at elevated or febrile body temperatures. For example, the virus responsible for "fever blisters," herpes simplex, is a frequent complication of many febrile diseases (Fenner et al. 1974). It is not known, however, whether the growth of these viruses is facilitated by the increased temperature or by some other aspect of the febrile episode.

Many species of bacteria are known to have their growth inhibited by febrile temperatures. For example, some strains of pneumococci are killed outright by temperatures as low as 41° to 41.5°C (Bennett and Nicastri 1960). In fact, Enders and Schaffer (1936) and others have shown that the virulence of pneumococci infections in rabbits paralleled their ability to grow in cultures at 41°C. Since rabbits normally maintain an afebrile body temperature of about 39.5°C and often reach body temperatures of 41° to 42°C during infections, this seems to be a case where an elevation in body temperature increases the survival rate by a direct effect on the microorganisms.

Gonococci are another group of bacteria which are particularly sensitive to elevations in temperature. Carpenter et al. (1933) found that temperatures of 40° to 41°C killed gonococci and this gave support to the then popular use of fever as a therapeutic agent in the treatment of gonorrhea.

The spirochetes responsible for causing neurosyphilis are also killed by elevations in temperature, although these elevations must be over 41°C (Bruetsch 1949). Bruetsch reviewed the evidence for the beneficial effects of malarial-induced fevers and concluded that since malarial fevers seldom reached 41°C, the direct effect of temperature on these organisms was only a minor factor. Apparently, several aspects of the host defense mechanisms are enhanced in response to malarial infections.

The in vitro growth of *A. hydrophila* is depressed by about

40% at temperatures of 42°C, compared to that at 34° to 40°C (Kluger et al. 1975). It would seem that the increase in survival of *A. hydrophila*-infected lizards held at 40°C was not related to a direct effect of temperature on the growth of these bacteria; however, the further increase in survival rate in lizards held at 42°C might well be related to the direct effect of temperature on these bacteria.

It is also possible that in vitro determinations of growth of microorganisms might not accurately reflect what is happening in vivo. For example, serum iron and zinc levels fall and serum copper levels generally rise during infection (see reviews in Beisel et al. 1974; Bullen et al. 1974; Weinberg 1978). It has been suggested by Weinberg (1974) and by others that the fall in serum iron, and perhaps zinc, might reduce the growth of pathogenic microorganisms. In fact, many studies have shown that certain species of bacteria grow poorly in a medium containing low levels of iron and that iron supplements increase the growth of bacteria in vitro and in vivo (Bullen et al. 1974; Kochan 1977). This exciting new area of immunology has been termed "nutritional immunity" by Kochan (1973).

Garibaldi (1972) has shown that the ability of *Salmonella typhimurium* to produce iron transport compounds (siderophores) is diminished by small elevations in temperature, and as a result it has been suggested that the reduction in serum iron, coupled with an elevation in body temperature (fever), is a coordinated host defense mechanism (Garibaldi 1972; Weinberg 1974). (To further support this contention, it has recently been shown that the leukocyte derived protein which is responsible for the fall in serum iron ["leukocyte endogenous mediator"] and for the development of fever [endogenous pyrogens] is probably the same compound (Merriman et al. 1977; Klempner et al. 1978.)

In order to attempt to relate changes in serum (or plasma) iron to fever and disease, Grieger and Kluger (1977 & 1978) studied the effects of bacterial infection on serum iron in desert iguanas. They found that during infection with *A. hydrophila* the serum iron levels of these lizards fell by about 30%. This fall was not directly related to the lizard's body temperature. When *A. hydrophila* were grown in vitro, there was little difference in the rate of growth at the normal (38°C) and febrile (41°C) temperatures when the iron concentrations of the growth media were maintained at the physiological levels found in uninfected lizards. However, a reduction in the available iron levels by precipitation (with $MgCO_3$) or by chelation (adding desferrioxamine B-sulphate) led to marked reductions in the growth rate of the bacteria at 41°C but not at 38°C. These data were interpreted to support the above hypothesis that one of the mechanisms behind fever's adaptive function is to decrease the pathogenic bacteria's ability to sequester adequate amounts of iron for normal growth.

Similar results have been found in rabbits during infection with *P. multocida* (Kluger and Rothenburg 1979). During infection, the plasma iron concentration of rabbits fell from 261 μg Fe/100 ml plasma to 66 μg Fe/100 ml plasma. During this time, these rabbits developed a fever. When the pathogenic bacteria were grown in vitro in a medium containing these reduced levels of iron, they grew well only at the afebrile temperatures. At the moderate febrile temperature of 41°C, the growth of the bacteria was inhibited by the low iron content. The growth of the bacteria was identical at the afebrile and febrile temperatures when the iron content approximated the normal uninfected levels.

It is likely that changes in other essential minerals and nutrients in the body fluids of infected animals also contribute to their survival. Whether these changes result in temperature dependent decreases in the growth of these pathogenic organisms (as in the cases of *A. hydrophila* and of *P. multocida* and iron levels) remains to be determined.

B. Effect of Temperature on the Host Defense Mechanisms

In addition to the direct effect of temperature on the growth potential of pathogenic organisms, there are undoubtedly many host defense mechanisms which are enhanced by higher temperatures. One area which has received considerable attention is that of antibody formation. Bennett and

Nicastri (1960) reviewed the literature concerning fever and antibody production and concluded that "any advantage that fever might give a host in producing antibody is likely to be offset by the enhanced pathogenicity of the infecting organism." They go on to caution, however, that "the data are too sparse to permit generalization and are useful only as a signal to caution in drawing sweeping conclusions." It seems likely that since it often takes days for antibody levels to rise following initial contact with a pathogen, that increased antibody production at febrile body temperatures would probably have, at best, a minor role as a host defense mechanism.

Another aspect of the immune response which is thought to be affected by temperature is lysosome function. Recall that lysosomes are intracellular particles containing large amounts of hydrolytic enzymes which are capable of breaking down or digesting many substances. It is thought that one of the reasons that tumor cells are more readily killed by heat (when compared to nonmalignant cells) is that the lysosomal membrane in the tumor cells is more heat sensitive (Overgaard 1977). As a result, the digestive enzymes are more easily liberated, resulting in the destruction of these cells. Lysosomes in normal cells, however, are also thought to be somewhat sensitive to heat.

Lwoff (1969) has hypothesized that one of the reasons fever is beneficial during viral infections is that elevations in body temperature, combined with the effects of viruses on lysosomes, increase lysosomal lesions. This liberates the lysosomal enzymes and results in the death of the virus and often the cell (autolysis). Lwoff suggests that "lysosomes are generally considered to be part of the suicidal machinery of the cell. . . . However, the fact that lysosomal enzymes may kill the cell is not in contradiction with their useful role during viral infection. The liberation of lysosomal enzymes, despite the fact that it kills the infected cell, could be an efficient defense mechanism against the virus. The death of a cell is sometimes beneficial for the organism." As such, the liberation of the lysosomal enzymes, triggered in part by an elevation in body temperature, might be one of the mechanisms behind fever's adaptive function.

Interferons are another group of proteins whose production is thought to be increased by elevated temperatures. These proteins are produced by many different cell types in response to intracellular contact with various foreign substances, most notably viruses. The entry of these activating agents into interferon-producing cells induces the production of interferons which are then secreted by these cells, resulting in the nonspecific inhibition of the growth and synthesis of many types of viruses.

In 1970, Ho reviewed the literature concerning the effects of temperature on the production of interferons and concluded that "the stimulation of interferon by viruses is inhibited by low temperatures, and there is some suggestion that the optimum temperature for interferon production is somewhat higher than that for replication of viruses." It is, to my knowledge, currently unknown whether small elevations in in vivo temperature, simulating normal 2° or 3°C fevers, increase the production of interferons.

Lymphocyte transformation is also thought to be enhanced by elevations in temperature. Lymphocytes are specialized types of leukocytes which are responsible for cellular and humoral immunity. In response to various stimulants or activators, these cells undergo proliferation and transformation and as a result are then capable of participating in various aspects of the immune response. It has recently been shown that temperatures corresponding to moderate fevers in human beings (38.5° to 39.0°C) result in an enhancement and an acceleration of lymphocyte transformation in response to various types of antigens (Roberts and Steigbigel 1977; Ashman and Nahmias 1977).

Another, and perhaps the most important, component of the immune response involves the role of polymorphonuclear granulocytes. It is the function of these white blood cells to reach the site of infection and to ingest and then digest the foreign substances.

There is some evidence that the mobility of these cells is increased with increasing temperature. Bryant et al. (1966) showed that the in vitro migration of leukocytes increased as the temperature was raised from 20° to 40°C. Similar findings were reported by Nahas et al. (1971). In this study they found that in human polymorphonuclear neutrophils the greatest increase in movement occurred between 35° and 40°C (Figure 48). The Q_{10} for the movement of these white blood cells was 5.2 between 32° and 42°C. Phelps and Stanislaw (1969) also found great increases in the mobility of white blood cells between 34° and 38°C; however, there was little increase between 37° and 38.5°C. Overall, these in vitro data are in agreement with the in vivo data reported by Bernheim et al. (1978) for the movement of granulocytes in desert iguanas.

Another aspect of leukocyte function that could be affected by temperature is its phagocytic activity. In 1942, Ellingson and Clark reported that, in vitro, human leukocytes ingested more bacteria at febrile temperatures between 38°

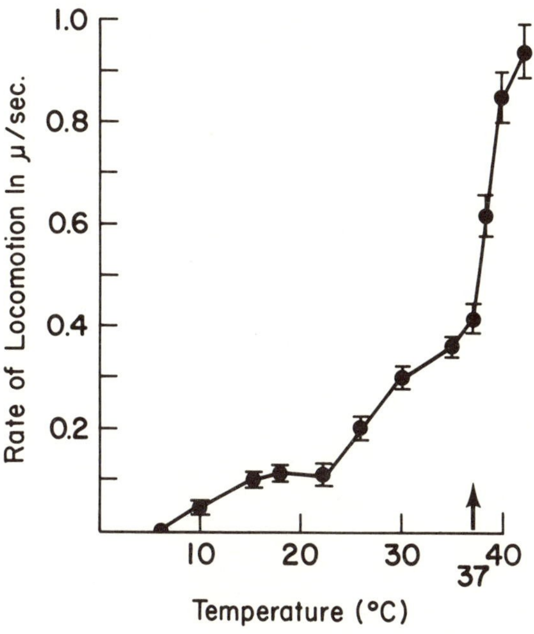

Figure 48. The rate of locomotion of human polymorphonuclear granulocytes as a function of temperature. (From Nahas et al. 1971.)

and 42°C than at afebrile temperatures. These results, however, have not been confirmed by others. For example, both Mandel (1975) and Sebag et al. (1977) have reported that there were no differences in polymorphonuclear phagocytic activity between afebrile and febrile temperatures.

Not only must white blood cells ingest the pathogenic organisms, they must also digest or kill them. Sebag et al. (1977) noted that elevations in temperature led to increased killing of some species of bacteria but had little effect on others. Craig and Suter (1966) reported that the percent of ingested staphylococcus bacteria which were killed increased as the temperature was raised from 26°C to 36°C; however, above 36°C this percentage remained fairly constant. Therefore, they suggested that fever does not increase intracellular killing, since most fevers in human beings range between 38° and 40°C. This is not technically correct. While it is true that the average rectal temperature of a febrile person might be between 38° and 40°C, the average body temperature might only range between 36° and 37°C. This is because the average body temperature incorporates both the warmer deep body areas and the cooler peripheral areas (skin, respiratory tract, limbs, etc.). Since many infections reside in areas cooler than found deep within the body, an increase in intracellular killing by white blood cells at 36°C might still represent a beneficial effect of fever. Our current understanding of the mechanisms behind the adaptive value of fever is summarized in Figure 49.

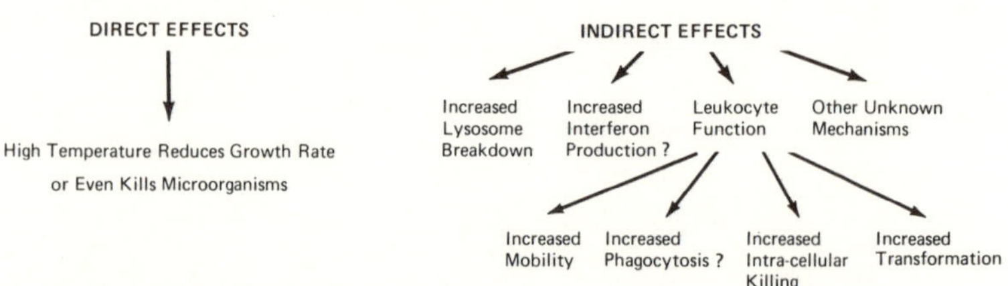

Figure 49. The mechanisms behind the adaptive value of fever.

Summary

Historically, fever has been considered to have an adaptive function. From the time of Hippocrates, about 2,400 years ago, to that of Liebermeister in the late 1800s, moderate fevers were looked upon as aiding the host organism in overcoming infection; however, proof of a beneficial function for fever had been lacking.

One type of observation which has been used to support an adaptive role for fever was that of fever therapy. Although fever therapy apparently has practical value in combating various types of infections, it clearly does not relate to naturally occurring fevers and therefore cannot legitimately be used to support, or refute, an adaptive role for fever.

Studies on mammals involving the correlation of fever with mortality (Vaughn and Kluger 1977) or morbidity (Toms et al. 1977) suggested that fever was beneficial. These studies, however, are difficult to interpret. Antipyretic studies have been even more difficult to interpret, with one (Klastersky 1971) suggesting that fever was harmful and another (Vaughn and Kluger 1977) that fever was beneficial. The results of hypothermia and hyperthermia have also led to mixed results; however, based on studies involving newborns, these types of studies have supported an adaptive role for fever in disease (Haahr and Mogensen 1977).

The use of the comparative method has led to results which are more easily interpreted. The fact that fever occurs in vertebrates from fishes through mammals is by itself a fairly convincing argument that fever has an adaptive function. It is unlikely that a process which is so energetically costly would be such a common occurrence during infection if it had no beneficial role. Furthermore, specific studies designed to answer the question of whether fever was adaptive or maladaptive using reptiles and fishes have shown that fever has survival value in reptiles (Kluger et al. 1975; Bernheim and Kluger 1976b) and in fishes (Covert and Reynolds 1977).

Overall, fever appears to have an adaptive value. The implication of this finding is that perhaps rather than attempting to attenuate fevers of moderate levels in patients, fevers should be allowed to run their course. Clearly, antipyretic drugs should be used with discretion. At times, it might even be advantageous to raise moderate fevers to somewhat higher levels. Obviously, more work needs to be done to specifically determine when, and for what types of infections, fever is beneficial.

The mechanisms behind fever's adaptive role can be divided into two categories—the direct and indirect effects of increased temperature. Many microorganisms are killed by elevations in temperature corresponding to moderate fevers (see Bennett and Nicastri 1960). One area which has recently begun to receive some attention is that of nutritional immunity. For example, in response to many types of pathogenic organisms, plasma or serum iron levels (as well as concentrations of some other nutrients) fall. Whereas the growth of certain species of pathogenic bacteria is not diminished by febrile temperatures when iron levels are high, these bacteria might not grow as rapidly at febrile temperatures when iron levels are lowered. This might be one of the mechanisms behind the beneficial effect of fever in lizards infected with *A. hydrophila* (Grieger and Kluger 1978).

An elevation in body temperature also indirectly affects the immune response. It does not appear that differences between serum antibody levels at afebrile and febrile temperatures have a major role in the survival value of fever. One possibly beneficial effect of elevated temperature is, however, an increased susceptibility of lysosomes to breakage, resulting in the death of viruses within the cell. The lysosomal enzymes digest the virus, and often the cell itself, resulting in a potentially effective host defense mechanism against viral infections.

Another beneficial effect of elevated or febrile temperatures involves white blood cell functions. Lymphocytes seem to undergo increased transformation and polymorphonuclear granulocytes appear to be more mobile at higher temperatures. Whereas the ability of these granulocytes to phagocytize foreign particles is not substantially changed, in some cases small elevations in temperature allow them to more readily kill the engulfed microorganisms.

Undoubtedly, many other aspects of the host's immunological repertoire will be found to be affected by increases in temperature. Some of these will be found to function more efficiently and others less efficiently at febrile body temperatures, with the net result that of generally increasing the host's defenses against pathogenic microorganisms. Overall, it appears that we are on the verge of verifying Sydenham's belief that "fever is Nature's engine which she brings into the field to remove her enemy."

References

Adler, R. D., and R.J.T. Joy. 1965. Febrile responses to the intracisternal injection of endogenous (leucocytic) pyrogen in the rabbit. *Soc. Exp. Biol. Med., Proc.* 119:660-663.

Adler, R. D., M. D. Rawlins, C. Rosendorff, and W. I. Cranston. 1969. The effect of salicylate on pyrogen-induced fever in man. *Clin. Sci.* 37:91-97.

Allen, I. V. 1965. The cerebral effects of endogenous serum and granulocytic pyrogen. *Brit. J. Exptl. Pathol.* 46:25-34.

Allen, J. A., and I. C. Roddie. 1972. The role of circulating catecholamines in sweat production in man. *J. Physiol.* (Lond.) 227:801-814.

Altman, P. L., and D. S. Dittmer, eds. (1974). Vol. III *Biology Data Book*, 2nd ed. *Fed. Amer. Soc. Exp. Biol.*

Ambache, N., H. C. Brummer, J. G. Rose, and J. Whiting. 1966. Thin-layer chromatography of spasmogenic unsaturated hydroxyacids from various tissues. *J. Physiol.* (Lond.) 185:77-78P.

Amend, D. F. 1970. Control of infectious hematopoietic necrosis virus disease by elevating the water temperature. *J. Fish. Res. Board Can.* 27:265-270.

———. 1976. Prevention and control of viral diseases of salmonids. *J. Fish. Res. Board Can.* 33:1059-1066.

Andersson, B., C. C. Gale, B. Hokfelt, and B. Larson. 1965. Acute and chronic effects of preoptic lesions. *Acta Physiol. Scand.* 65:45-60.

Artunkal, A. A., and E. Marley. 1974. Hyper- and hypothermic effects of prostaglandin E_1 (PGE_1) and their potentiation by indomethacin, in chicks. *J. Physiol.* (Lond.) 242:141-142P.

Ashman, R. B., and A. J. Nahmias. 1977. Enhancement of human lymphocyte responses to phytomitogens in vitro by incubation at elevated temperatures. *Clin. exp. Immunol.* 29:464-467.

Atkins, E., and P. Bodel. 1972. Fever. *New England J. Med.* 286:27-34.

———. 1974. Fever. In *The inflammatory process*, 2nd ed., ed. B. W. Zweifach, L. Grant, and R. T. McCluskey. Vol. III, pp. 467-514. New York: Academic Press.

Atkins, E., M. Cronin, and P. Isacson. 1964. Endogenous pyrogen release from rabbit blood cells incubated in vitro with parainfluenza virus. *Science* 146:1469-1470.

Atkins, E., and L. Francis. 1977. Additional studies on the role of a lymphokine in the genesis of antigen-induced fever in delayed hypersensitivity. In *Drugs, Biogenic Amines and Body Temperature*. 3rd Symp. of the Pharmacology of Thermoregulation, ed. K. E. Cooper, P. Lomax, and E. Schonbaum. pp. 118-121. Basel: S. Karger.

Atkins, E., and L. R. Freedman. 1963. Studies in staphylococcal fever. I. Responses to bacterial cells. *Yale J. Biol. Med.* 63:451-471.

Atkins, E., and W. C. Huang. 1958. Studies on the pathogenesis of fever with influenza viruses. *J. Expt. Med.* 107:383-401.

Atkins, E., and W. B. Wood, Jr. 1955. Studies on the pathogenesis of fever. I. The presence of transferable pyrogen in the blood stream following the injection of typhoid vaccine. *J. Expt. Med.* 101:519-528.

Atwood, R. P., and E. H. Kass. 1964. Relationship of body temperature to the lethal action of bacterial endotoxin. *J. Clin. Invest.* 43:151-159.

Avery, D. D., and P. E. Penn. 1974. Blockage of pyrogen induced fever by intrahypothalamic injections of salicylate in the rat. *Neuropharm.* 13:1179-1185.

Baird, J. A., J.R.S. Hales, and W. J. Lang. 1974. Thermoregulatory responses to the injection of monamines, acetylcholine and prostaglandins into a lateral cerebral ventricle of the echidna. *J. Physiol.* (Lond.) 236:539-548.

Bakker, R. T. 1975. Experimental and fossil evidence for the evolution of tetrapod bioenergetics. In *Perspectives of Biophysical Ecology*, ed. D. M. Gates and R. B. Schmerl, pp. 365-399. New York: Springer-Verlag.

Bakker, R. T., and P. G. Galton. 1974. Dinosaur monophyly and a new class of vertebrates. *Nature* 248:168-172.

Bang, F. B. 1956. A bacterial disease of Limulus polyphemus. *Bull. Johns Hopkins Hosp.* 98:325-351.

Barber, M. A. 1908. The rate of multiplication of *Bacillus coli* at different temperatures. *J. Infect. Dis.* 5:379-400.

Barrett, J. T. 1974. Textbook of immunology, an introduction to immunochemistry and immunobiology. Saint Louis: C. V. Mosby Co.

Bartholomew, G. A. 1977. Body temperature and energy

metabolism. In *Animal Physiology, Principles and Adaptations*, ed. M. S. Gordon, pp. 364-449. New York: Macmillan Co.

Beeson, P. B. 1947a. Tolerance to bacterial pyrogens I. Factors influencing its development. *J. Expt. Med.* 86:29-38.

———. 1947b. Tolerance to bacterial pyrogens II. Role of the reticulo-endothelial system. *J. Expt. Med.* 86:39-44.

———. 1948. Observations on the fever caused by bacterial pyrogens I. A study of the relationship between the fever caused by bacterial pyrogens and the fever accompanying acute infections. *J. Expt. Med.* 88:267-278.

Beisel, W. R., R. S. Pekarek, and R. W. Wannemacher, Jr. 1974. The impact of infectious disease on trace-element metabolism of the host. In *Trace Element Metabolism in Animals*, ed. W. G. Hoekstra, J. W. Suttie, H. E. Ganther, and W. Mertz, pp. 217-240. Baltimore: University Park Press.

Benacerraf, B., M. M. Sebestyen, and S. Schlossman. 1959. A quantitative study of the kinetics of blood clearance of P^{32}-labelled *Escherichia coli* and staphylococci by the reticuloendothelial system. *J. Expt. Med.* 110:27-48.

Bennett, I. L., Jr., and P. B. Beeson. 1950. The properties and biologic effects of bacterial pyrogens. *Medicine* (Balt.) 29:365-400.

———. 1953a. Studies on the pathogenesis of fever I. The effect of injection of extracts and suspensions of uninfected rabbit tissues upon the body temperature of normal rabbits. *J. Expt. Med.* 98:477-492.

———. 1953b. Studies on the pathogenesis of fever II. Characterization of fever-producing substances from polymorphonuclear leukocytes and from the fluid of sterile exudates. *J. Expt. Med.* 98:493-508.

Bennett, I. L., Jr., and L. E. Cluff. 1952. Influence of nitrogen mustard upon reactions to bacterial endotoxins: Shwartzman phenomenon and fever. *Proc. Soc. Exp. Biol.* N.Y. 81:304-307.

———. 1957. Bacterial pyrogens. *Pharm. Rev.* 9:427-475.

Bennett, I. L., Jr., and A. Nicastri. 1960. Fever as a mechanism of resistance. *Bact. Rev.* 24:16-34.

Bennett, I. L., Jr., R. R. Wagner, and V. S. LeQuire. 1949. The production of fever by influenza virus. II. Tolerance in rabbits to the pyrogenic effect of influenza viruses. *J. Expt. Med.* 90:335-347.

Benzinger, T. H. 1977. *Temperature*, Part 1, Arts and Concepts. Stroudsburg, Pa.: Dowden, Hutchinson and Ross, Inc.

Berk, M. L., and J. E. Heath. 1976. Effects of preoptic, hypothalamic, and telencephalic lesions on thermoregulation in the lizard, *Dipsosaurus dorsalis*. *J. Therm. Biol.* 1:65-78.

Bernheim, H. A., P. T. Bodel, P. Askenase, and E. Atkins. 1978. Effects of fever on host defence mechanisms after infection in the lizard *Dipsosaurus dorsalis*. *Br. J. exp. Path.* 59:76-84.

Bernheim, H. A., and M. J. Kluger. 1976a. Fever and antipyresis in the lizard *Dipsosaurus dorsalis*. *Am. J. Physiol.* 231:198-203.

———. 1976b. Fever: effect of drug-induced antipyresis on survival. *Science* 193:237-239.

———. 1977. Endogenous pyrogen-like substance produced by reptiles. *J. Physiol.* (Lond.) 267:659-666.

Birkebak, R. C. 1966. Heat transfer in biological systems. *Int'l. Rev. of Gen. and Exp. Zool.* 2:269-344.

Blair, W. F., A. P. Blair, P. Brodkorb, F. R. Cagle, and G. A. Moore. 1957. *Vertebrates of the United States*. New York: McGraw-Hill.

Bligh, J. 1973. *Temperature regulation in mammals and other vertebrates*. Amsterdam: North-Holland Publ. Co.

Bodel, P. 1970. Studies on the mechanism of endogenous pyrogen production. I. Investigation of new protein synthesis in stimulated human blood leucocytes. *Yale J. Biol. Med.* 43:145-163.

———. 1974. Tumors and fever. Part I. Generalized pertubations in host physiology caused by localized tumors. *Annals of N.Y. Acad. Sci.* 230:6-13.

Bodel, P., and E. Atkins. 1966. Human leukocyte pyrogen producing fever in rabbits. *Soc. Exp. Biol. Med., Proc.* 121:943-946.

Bodel, P., C. R. Reynolds, and E. Atkins. 1973. Lack of effect of salicylate on pyrogen release from human blood leucocytes in vitro. *Yale J. Biol. Med.* 46:190-195.

Bolton, H. C. 1900. *Evolution of the Thermometer: 1592-1743*. Easton: Chemical Publ.

Bornstein, D. L., C. Bredenberg, and W. B. Wood, Jr. 1963. Studies on the pathogenesis of fever. XI. Quantitative features of the febrile response to leucocytic pyrogen. *J. Expt. Med.* 117:349-364.

Bornstein, D. L., and J. W. Woods. 1969. Species specificity of leukocyte pyrogens. *J. Expt. Med.* 130:707-721.

Boulant, J. A., and J. D. Hardy. 1974. The effect of spinal and skin temperature on the firing rate and thermosensitivity of preoptic neurones. *J. Physiol.* (Lond.) 240:639-660.

Bourn, J. M., and F. B. Seibert. 1925. The cause of many febrile reactions following intravenous injections II. The bacteriology of twelve distilled waters. *Am. J. Physiol.* 71:652-659.

Brattsrom, B. 1970. Amphibia. In *Comparative Physiology of Thermoregulation*, ed. G. C. Whittow, pp. 135-166. New York: Academic Press.

Brengelmann, G. 1973. Temperature Regulation. In *Physiology and Biophysics*, ed. T. C. Ruch and H. D. Patton, pp. 105-135. Philadelphia: W. B. Saunders Co.

Bruetsch, W. L. 1949. Why malaria cures general paralysis. *Indiana State Med. Assoc. J.* 42:211-216.

Bryant, R. E., R. M. DesPrez, M. H. VanWay, and D. E. Rogers. 1966. Studies on human leukocyte motility I. Effects of alterations in pH, electrolyte concentration, and phagocytosis on leukocyte migration, adhesiveness, and aggregation. *J. Expt. Med.* 124:483-499.

Bryden, D. J. 1971. An additional factor in the history of the centigrade thermometer. *Brit. J. for Hist. Sci.* 5:393-396.

Bullen, J. J., H. J. Rogers, and E. Griffiths. 1974. Bacterial iron metabolism and immunity. In *Microbial Iron Metabolism, A Comprehensive Treatise,* ed. J. B. Neilands, pp. 517-551. New York: Academic Press.

Cabanac, M., R. Duclaux, and A. Gillet. 1970. Thermoregulation comportementale chez le chien: effets de la fievre et la thyroxine. *Physiol. and Behavior*. 5:697-704.

Cabanac, M., and B. Massonnet. 1974. Temperature regulation during fever: change of set point or change of gain? A tentative answer from a behavioral study in man. *J. Physiol.* (Lond.) 238:561-568.

Cabanac, M., J.A.J. Stolwijk, and J. D. Hardy. 1968. Effect of temperature and pyrogens on single-unit activity in the rabbit's brain stem. *J. Appl. Physiol.* 24:645-652.

Carey, F. G., and K. D. Lawson. 1973. Temperature regulation in free-swimming bluefin tuna. *Comp. Biochem. Physiol.* 44:375-392.

Carey, F. G., and J. M. Teal. 1969. Mako and porbeagle: warm-bodied sharks. *Comp. Biochem. Physiol.* 28:199-204.

Carlson, L. D., and A.C.L. Hsieh. 1970. *Control of energy exchange*. New York: Macmillan Co.

Carmichael, L. E., F. D. Barnes, and D. H. Percy. 1969. Temperature as a factor in resistance of young puppies. *J. Infect. Dis.* 120:669-678.

Carpenter, C. M., R. A. Boak, L. A. Mucci, and S. L. Warren. 1933. Studies on the physiologic effects of fever temperatures. The thermal death time of *Neisseria gonorrhoeae* in vitro with special reference to fever temperatures. *J. Lab. Clin. Med.* 18:981-990.

Casterlin, M. E., and W. W. Reynolds. 1977a. Behavioral fever in anuran amphibian larvae. *Life Sci.* 20:593-596.

———. 1977b. Behavioral fever in crayfish. *Hydrobiologia* 56:99-101.

Cavaliere, R., E. C. Ciocatto, B. C. Giovanella, C. Heidelberger, R. O. Johnson, M. Margottini, B. Mondovi, G. Moricca, and A. Rossi-Fanelli. 1967. Selective heat sensitivity of cancer cells. *Cancer* 20:1351-1381.

Chai, C. Y. and S. C. Wang. 1970. Cardiovascular and respiratory responses to cooling to the medulla oblongata of the cat. *Soc. Exp. Biol. and Med., Proc.* 134:763-767.

Church, N. S. 1960. Heat loss and the body temperatures of flying insects II. Heat conduction within the body and its loss by radiation and convection. *J. Expt. Biol.* 37:186-212.

Clark, W. G. 1970. The antipyretic effects of acetaminophen and sodium salicylate on endotoxin-induced fevers in cats. *J. Pharmacol. Exp. Ther.* 175:469-475.

———. 1971. Hyperthermic effect of disodium edetate injected into the lateral ventricle of the unanesthetized cat. *Experientia* 27:1452-1454.

Clark, W. G., and H. R. Cumby. 1975. The antipyretic effect of indomethacin. *J. Physiol.* (Lond.) 248:625-638.

Clark, W. G., and S. G. Moyer. 1972. The effects of acetaminophen and sodium salicylate on the release and activity of leukocytic pyrogen in the cat. *J. Pharmacol. Exp. Ther.* 181:183-191.

Colbert, E. H. 1961. Evolution of the vertebrates. New York: Wiley and Sons, Inc.

Connor, D. G., and E. H. Kass. 1961. Effect of artificial fever in increasing susceptibility to bacterial endotoxin. *Nature* (Lond.) 190:453-454.

Cooper, K. E., W. I. Cranston, and E. S. Snell. 1964. Temperature regulation during fever in man. *Clin. Sci.* 27:345-356.

Cooper, K. E., W. I. Cranston, and A. J. Honour. 1967. Observations on the site and mode of action of pyrogens in the rabbit brain. *J. Physiol.* (Lond.) 191:325-337.

Cooper, K. E., and W. L. Veale. 1972. The effect of injecting an inert oil into the cerebral ventricular system upon fever produced by intravenous leucocyte pyrogen. *Can. J. Physiol. Pharm.* 11:1066-1071.

Covert, J. B., and W. W. Reynolds. 1977. Survival value of fever in fish. *Nature* 267:43-45.

Cowles, R. B. 1958. Possible origin of dermal temperature regulation. *Evolution* 12:347-357.

Cox, B., and P. Lomax. 1977. Pharmacologic control of temperature regulation. *Ann. Rev. Pharmacol. Toxicol.* 17:341-353.

Coxe, J. R. 1846. *The writings of Hippocrates and Galen*. Philadelphia: Lindsay and Blakiston.

Craig, C. P., and E. Suter. 1966. Extracellular factors influencing staphylocidal capacity of human polymorphonuclear leukocytes. *J. Immunol.* 97:287-296.

Cranston, W. I., R. F. Hellon, and D. Mitchell. 1975. A dissociation between fever and prostaglandin concentration in cerebrospinal fluid. *J. Physiol.* (Lond.) 253:583-592.

Cranston, W. I., R. H. Luff, M. D. Rawlins, and C. Rosendorff. 1970. The effects of salicylate on temperature regulation in the rabbit. *J. Physiol.* (Lond.) 208:251-259.

Crawford, E. C., Jr., and B. J. Barber. 1974. Effects of core, skin, and brain temperature on panting in the lizard *Sauromalus obesus*. *Am. J. Physiol.* 226:569-573.

D'Alecy, L. G., and M. J. Kluger. 1975. Avian febrile response. *J. Physiol.* (Lond.) 253:223-232.

Dascombe, M. J. 1976. Studies on the possible involvement of adenosine 3′-5′-monophosphate in thermoregulation during fever. Ph.D. thesis, Aberdeen.

Davson, H. 1970. *Physiology of the cerebrospinal fluid*. London: J. & A. Churchill.

Dawson, T. J., D. Robertshaw, and C. R. Taylor. 1974. Sweating in the kangaroo: a cooling mechanism during exercise, but not in the heat. *Am. J. Physiol.* 227:494-498.

Dawson, W. R., and J. W. Hudson. 1970. Birds. In *Comparative Physiology of Thermoregulation*, ed. G. C. Whittow, pp. 224-310. New York: Academic Press.

Desmond, A. J. 1975. *The hot-blooded dinosaurs: a revolution in palaeontology*. New York: Dial Press.

Dinarello, C. A., P. Bodel, and E. Atkins. 1968. The role of the liver in production of fever and in pyrogenic tolerance. *Trans. Assoc. Amer. Phys.* 81:334-344.

Dinarello, C. A., N. P. Goldin, and S. M. Wolff. 1974. Demonstration and characterization of two distinct human leukocytic pyrogens. *J. Expt. Med.* 139:1369-1381.

Dinarello, C. A., L. Renfer, and S. M. Wolff. Human leukocytic pyrogen: purification and development of a radioimmunoassay. *Proc. Nat'l. Acad. Sci.* U.S.A. 74:4624-4627, 1977.

Douglas, W. W. 1975. Polypeptides-angiotensin, plasma kinins, and other vasoactive agents; prostaglandins. In *The Pharmacological*

Basis of Therapeutics, ed. L. S. Goodman and A. Gilman. New York: Macmillan Co.

Dubois, E. F. 1948. Fever and the regulation of body temperature. Springfield: C. C. Thomas.

Duclaux, R., M. Fantino, and M. Cabanac. 1973. Comportement thermoregulateur chez *Rana esculenta. Pflugers Arch.* 342:347-358.

Duran-Reynals, M. L. 1946. The fever bark tree: the pageant of quinine. New York: Doubleday and Co., Inc.

Eisenman, J. S. 1969. Pyrogen-induced changes in the thermosensitivity of septal and preoptic neurons. *Am. J. Physiol.* 216:330-334.

Ellingson, H. V., and P. F. Clark. 1942. The influence of artificial fever on mechanisms of resistance. *J. Immunol.* 43:65-83.

Ellis, P. P., and D. L. Smith 1973. *Handbook of Ocular Therapeutics and Pharmacology*. 4th ed. St. Louis: Mosby.

Enders, J. F., and M. F. Shaffer. 1936. Studies on natural immunity to pneumococcus type III. I. The capacity of strains of pneumococcus type III to grow at 41°C and their virulence for rabbits. *J. Expt. Med.* 64:7-18.

Farr, R. S., D. H. Campbell, S. L. Clark, Jr., and J. E. Proffitt. 1954a. The febrile response of sensitized rabbits to the intravenous injection of antigen. *Anat. Rec.* 118:385-386.

Farr, R. S., S. L. Clark, Jr., J. E. Proffitt, and D. H. Campbell. 1954b. Some humoral aspects of the development of tolerance to bacterial pyrogens in rabbits. *Am. J. Physiol.* 177:269-278.

Favorite, G. O., and H. R. Morgan. 1942. Effects produced by the intravenous injection in man of a toxic antigenic material derived from *Eberthella typhosa*: clinical, hematological, chemical and seratological studies. *J. Clin. Invest.* 21:589-599.

Feldberg, W., K. P. Gupta, A. S. Milton, and S. Wendlandt. 1973. Effect of pyrogen and antipyretics on prostaglandin activity in cisternal c.s.f. of unanesthetized cats. *J. Physiol.* (Lond.) 234:279-303.

Feldberg, W., R. D. Myers, and W. L. Veale. 1970. Perfusion from cerebral ventricle to cisterna magna in the unanesthetized cat. Effect of calcium on body temperature. *J. Physiol.* (Lond.) 207:403-416.

Feldberg, W., and P. N. Saxena. 1971. Further studies on prostaglandin E_1 fever in cats. *J. Physiol.* (Lond.) 219:739-745.

———. 1975. Prostaglandins, endotoxins and lipid A on body temperature in rats. *J. Physiol.* (Lond.) 249:601-615.

Feldberg, W. S., W. L. Veale, and K. E. Cooper. 1971. Does leucocyte pyrogen enter the anterior hypothalamus via the cerebrospinal fluid? *Proc. of the Int'l. Union of Physiol. Sci.* IX:511.

Fenner, F., B. R. McAuslan, C. A. Mims, J. Sambrook, and D. O. White. 1974. The biology of animal viruses. New York: Academic Press.

Ferreira. S. H., S. Moncada, and J. R. Vane. 1971. Indomethacin and aspirin abolish prostaglandin release from the spleen. *Nature New Biology* 231:237-239.

Ford, D. M. 1974. A selective action of prostaglandin E_1 on hypothalamic neurones in the cat which respond to brain cooling. *J. Physiol.* (Lond.) 242:142-143P.

Fraenkel, G. S. and D. L. Gunn. 1961. The orientation of animals: kineses, taxes and compass reactions. New York: Dover Publ., Inc.

Freeman, B. M. 1966. The effects of cold, noradrenaline and adrenaline upon the oxygen consumption and carbohydrate metabolism of the young fowl (*Gallus domesticus*). *Comp. Biochem. Physiol.* 18:369-382.

Frey, M. V. 1895. Beitrage zur sinnesphysiologie der Haut. III. *Ber. Sachs. Ges. (Akad.) Wiss.* 47:166-184.

Gander, G. W., J. Chaffee, and F. Goodale. 1967. Studies on the antipyretic action of salicylates. *Soc. Exp. Biol. Med., Proc.* 126:205-209.

Garibaldi, J. A. 1972. Influence of temperature on the biosynthesis of iron transport compounds by *Salmonella typhimurium*. *J. Bact.* 110:262-265.

Gates, D. M. 1972. *Man and his environment: Climate*. New York: Harper and Row.

Giese, A. C. 1968. *Cell Physiology*. 3rd ed. Philadelphia: W. B. Saunders Co.

Gonzalez, R. R., M. J. Kluger, and J. D. Hardy. 1971. Partitional calorimetery of the New Zealand white rabbit at temperatures 5-35°C. *J. Appl. Physiol.* 31:728-734.

Good, R. A. and R. L. Varco. 1955. A clinical and experimental study of agammaglobulinemia. *The Journal-Lancet* (Minneapolis) 75:245-271.

Gorke, K., R. Necker, and W. Rautenberg. 1975. Neurophysiological investigations of spinal reflexes at different temperatures of the spinal cord in birds and reptiles. *Pflugers Arch.* 359:269-271.

Gray, J. 1928. The growth of fish. III. The effect of temperature. *Proc. Roy. Soc. Lond.*, B95:6-15.

Greenleaf, J. E., S. Kolzowski, K. Nazar, H. Kaciuba-Uscilko,

Z. Brzeninska, and A. Ziemba. 1976. Ion-osmotic hyperthermia during exercise in dogs. *Am. J. Physiol.* 230:74-79.

Greenway, C. V., and V. S. Murthy. 1971. Mesenteric vasoconstriction after endotoxin administration in cats pretreated with aspirin. *Br. J. Pharmacol.* 43:259-269.

Greisman, S. E., F. A. Carozzo, Jr., and J. D. Hills. 1963. Mechanisms of endotoxin tolerance. I. Relationship between tolerance and reticuloendothelial system phagocytic activity in the rabbit. *J. Expt. Med.* 117:663-674.

Greisman, S. E. and C. L. Woodward. 1970. Mechanism of endotoxin tolerance. VII. The role of the liver. *J. Immunol.* 105:1468-1476.

Grieger, T. A., and M. J. Kluger. 1977. Effects of bacteria and temperature on free serum iron levels in the lizard *Dipsosaurus dorsalis*. *Fed. Proc.* 20(4):37.

———. 1978. Fever and Survival: the role of serum iron. *J. Physiol.* (Lond.) 279:187-196.

Grollman, A. 1930. Physiological variations of the cardiac output in man. *Am. J. Physiol.* 95:263-273.

Haahr, S., and S. Mogensen. 1977. Function of fever. *The Lancet.* Vol. II, No. 8038:613.

Hahn, H. H., S. F. Cheuk, C.D.S. Elfenbein, and W. B. Wood, Jr. 1970. Studies on the pathogenesis of fever. XIX. Localization of pyrogen in granulocytes. *J. Expt. Med.* 131:701-709.

Hales, J.R.S., J. W. Bennett, J. A. Baird, and A. A. Fawcett. 1973. Thermoregulatory effects of prostaglandins E_1, E_2, $F_1\alpha$ and $F_2\alpha$ in the sheep. *Pflugers Arch.* 339:125-133.

Hall, C. H., Jr., and E. Atkins. 1959. Studies on tuberculin fever. I. The mechanism of fever in tuberculin hypersensitivity. *J. Expt. Med.* 109:339-359.

Hamberg, M., J. Svensson, and B. Samuelson. 1975. Thromboxanes: a new group of biologically active compounds derived from prostaglandin endoperoxides. *Proc. Nat'l. Acad. Sci.*, U.S.A. 72:2994-2998.

Hammel, H. T. 1968. Regulation of internal body temperature. *Ann. Rev. Physiol.* 30:641-710.

Hanegan, J. L., and B. A. Williams. 1973. Brain calcium: role in temperature regulation. *Science* 181:663-664.

Hart, J. S., and O. Z. Roy. 1967. Temperature regulation during flight in pigeons. *Amer. J. Physiol.* 213:1311-1316.

Haynes, R. C., Jr., and J. Larner. 1975. Adrenocorticotropic hormone; adrenocortical steroids and their synthetic analogs; inhibitors of adrenocortical steroid biosynthesis. In *The Phar-*

macological Basis of Therapeutics, ed. L. S. Goodman and A. Gilman, pp. 1472-1506. New York: Macmillan Co.

Hayward, J. S. and C. P. Lyman. 1967. Nonshivering heat production during arousal from hibernation and evidence for the contribution of brown fat. In *Mammalian Hibernation III*, ed. K. C. Fisher, A. R. Dawe, C. P. Lyman, E. Schonbaum, and F. E. South, Jr., pp. 346-355. New York: American Elsevier.

Heath, J. E. 1965. Temperature regulation and diurnal activity in horned lizards. *Univ. California Publ. Zool.* 64:97-136.

———. 1967. Temperature responses of the periodical "17-year" cicada, *Magicicada cassini* (Homoptera, Cicadidae). *Amer. Midland Nat.* 77:64-76.

———. 1968. The origins of thermoregulation. In *Evolution and Environment*, ed. E. T. Drake, pp. 259-278. New Haven and London: Yale Univ. Press.

Heath, J. E., and P. A. Adams. 1965. Temperature regulation in the sphinx moth during flight. *Nature* 205:309-310.

Heath, J. E, J. L. Hanegan, P. J. Wilkin, and M. S. Heath. 1971. Thermoregulation by heat production and behavior in insects. *J. de Physiol.* 63:267-270.

Heath, J. E., and P. J. Wilkin. 1970. Temperature responses of the desert cicada, *Diceroprocta apache* (Homoptera, Cicadidae). *Physiol. Zool.* 43:145-154.

Heinrich, B. 1974. Thermoregulation in endothermic insects. *Science* 185:747-756.

———. 1977. The physiology of exercise in the bumblebee. *Amer. Scientist* 65:455-465.

Hellon, R. F. 1970. The stimulation of hypothalamic neurones by changes in ambient temperature. *Pflugers Arch.* 321:56-66.

———. 1975. Monamines, pyrogens and cations: their action on central control of body temperature. *Pharm. Rev.* 26:289-321.

Hellstrom, B., and H. T. Hammel. 1967. Some characteristics of temperature regulation in the unanesthetized dog. *Am. J. Physiol.* 213:547-556.

Hensel, H. 1974. Thermoreceptors. *Annual Rev. of Physiol.* 36:233-249.

Hensel, H., K. H. Andres, and M. V. During. 1974. Structure and function of cold receptors. *Pflugers Arch.* 352:1-10.

Hensel, H., K. Bruck, and P. Raths. 1973. Homeothermic Organisms, in *Temperature and Life*, ed. H. Precht, J. Christophersen, H. Hensel, and W. Larcher. New York: Springer-Verlag.

Hensel, H., and K. Schafer. 1974. Effects of calcium on warm and cold receptors. *Pflugers Arch.* 352:87-90.

Herion, J. C., R. I. Walker, and J. G. Palmer. 1961. Endotoxin fever in granulocytopenic animals. *J. Expt. Med.* 113:1115-1125.

Hipskind, S. G., and W. S. Hunter. 1977. Thermoregulatory response to visceral thermal stimulation in unanesthetized cats. *The Physiologist* 20(4):43.

Hirschsohn, J., and H. Maendl. 1922. Studien zur dynamik der endovenosen injektion bei anwendung von kalkium. *Wien Arch. inn. Med.* 4:379-414.

Ho, M. 1970. Factors influencing the interferon response. *Arch. Intern. Med.* 126:135-146.

Holmes, S. W., and E. W. Horton. 1968. The identification of four prostaglandins in the dog brain and their regional distribution in the central nervous system. *J. Physiol.* (Lond.) 195:731-741.

Hoo, S. L., M. T. Lin, R. D. Wei, C. Y. Chai, and S. C. Wang. 1972. Effects of sodium acetylsalicylate on the release of pyrogen from leukocytes. *Soc. Exp. Biol. Med., Proc.* 139:1155-1158.

Hort, E. C., and W. J. Penfold, 1911. The dangers of saline injections. *Brit. Med. Jour.* 2:1589-1591.

———. 1912. Microorganisms and their relation to fever. *J. Hyg.* (Lond.) 12:361-390.

Hull, D. 1971. Thermoregulation in Young Mammals. In *Comparative Physiology of Thermoregulation.* Vol. III. *Special aspects of thermoregulation*, ed. G. C. Whittow, pp. 167-200. New York: Academic Press.

Hutchison, V. H., H. G. Dowling, and A. Vinegar. 1966. Thermoregulation in a brooding female Indian python, *Python molurus bivittatus*. *Science* 151:694-696.

Jackson, D. L. 1967. A hypothalamic region responsive to localized injection of pyrogens. *J. Neurophysiol.* 30:586-602.

Jahanovsky, J. 1959. Demonstration of endogenous pyrogen in serum during systemic tuberculin reaction in rabbits. *Nature* (Lond.) 183:693-694.

Jansky, L. 1973. Non-shivering thermogenesis and its thermoregulatory significance. *Biol. Rev.* 48:85-132.

Jenkin, C. R., and D. Rowley. 1961. The role of opsonins in the clearance of living and inert particles by cells of reticuloendothelial system. *J. Expt. Med.* 114:363-374.

Jennings, H. S. 1906. *Behavior of the Lower Organisms*. New York: Columbia Univ. Press.

Jessen, C., and E. Th. Mayer. 1971. Spinal cord and hypothalamus as core sensors of temperature in the conscious dog. I. Equivalence of responses. *Pflugers Arch.* 324:189-204.

Johnson, F. H., H. Eyring, and M. J. Polissar. 1954. *The Kinetic Basis of Molecular Biology*. New York: Wiley and Sons, Inc.

Jones, W.H.S. 1923. Hippocrates (with an English translation). Vols. 1-4. New York: G. P. Putnam's Sons.

Kaiser, H. K., and W. B. Wood, Jr. 1962. Studies on the pathogenesis of fever. IX. The production of endogenous pyrogen by polymorphonuclear leucocytes. *J. Expt. Med.* 115:727-739.

Keller, A. D., and E. B. McClaskey. 1964. Localization, by the brain slicing method, of the level or levels of the cephalic brainstem upon which effective heat dissipation is dependent. *Am. J. of Physical Med.* 43:181-213.

King, M. K. 1964. Pathogenesis of fever in rabbits following intravenous injection of Coxsackie virus. *J. Lab. Clin. Med.* 63:23-29.

King, M. K., and W. B. Wood, Jr. 1958. Studies on the pathogenesis of fever. IV. The site of action of leucocytic and circulating endogenous pyrogen. *J. Expt. Med.* 107:291-303.

Klastersky, J. 1971. Etude experimentale et clinique des effets favorables et defavorables de la fievre et de l'administration de corticoides au cours d'infections bacteriennes. *Acta Clin. Belgica* 26 (Supplementun 6).

Klempner, M. S., C. A. Dinarello, and J. I. Gallin. 1978. Human leukocytic pyrogen induces release of specific granule contents from human neutrophils. *J. Clin. Invest.* 61:1330-1336.

Kluger, M. J. 1977. Fever in the frog *Hyla cinerea*. *J. Thermal Biol.* 2:79-81.

Kluger, M. J., R. R. Gonzalez, J. W. Mitchell, and J.A.J. Stolwijk. 1971. The rabbit ear as a temperature sensor. *Life Sciences* 10:895-899.

Kluger, M. J., R. R. Gonzalez, and J.A.J. Stolwijk. 1973a. Temperature regulation in the exercising rabbit. *Amer. J. Physiol.* 224:130-135.

Kluger, M. J., and J. E. Heath. 1970. Vasomotion in the bat wing: a thermoregulatory response to internal heating. *Comp. Biochem. Physiol.* 32:219-226.

———. 1971a. Thermoregulatory responses to preoptic-anterior hypothalamic heating and cooling in the bat, *Eptesicus fuscus*. *Z. vergl. Physiol.* 74:340-352.

———. 1971b. Effect of preoptic anterior hypothalamic lesions on thermoregulation in the bat. *Am. J. Physiol.* 221:144-419.

Kluger, M. J., D. H. Ringler, and M. R. Anver. 1975. Fever and survival. *Science* 188:166-168.

Kluger, M. J., and B. A. Rothenburg. 1979. Fever and reduced iron: their interaction as a host defense response to bacterial infection. *Science* 203:374-376.

Kluger, M. J., R. S. Tarr, and J. E. Heath. 1973b. Posterior hypothalamic lesions and disturbances in behavioral thermoregulation in the lizard *Dipsosaurus dorsalis*. *Physiol. Zool.* 46:79-84.

Kluger, M. J., and L. K. Vaughn. 1978. Fever and survival in rabbits infected with *Pasteurella multocida*. *J. Physiol.* (Lond.) 282:243-251.

Knight, H. C., M. L. Emory, and L. D. Flint. 1943. Method of inducing therapeutic fever with typhoid vaccine using intravenous drip technique. U. S. Public Health Service; *Venereal Dis. Inform*. 24:323-329.

Knutson, R. M. 1974. Heat production and temperature regulation in eastern skunk cabbage. *Science* 186:746-747.

Kochan, I. 1973. The role of iron in bacterial infections, with special consideration of host-tubercle Bacillus interaction. *Curr. Topics Micro. Immun.* 60:1-30.

———. 1977. Role of iron in the regulation of nutritional immunity. *Advan. In Chem. Ser.*, No. 162:55-77.

Kozak, M. S., H. H. Hahn, W. J. Lennarz, and W. B. Wood, Jr. 1968. Studies on the pathogenesis of fever. XVI. Purification and further characterization of granulocytic pyrogen. *J. Expt. Med.* 127:341-357.

Laburn, H., D. Mitchell, and C. Rosendorff. 1977. Effects of prostaglandin antagonism on sodium arachidonate fever in rabbits. *J. Physiol.* (Lond.) 267:559-570.

Levin, J., and F. B. Bang. 1964. The role of endotoxin in the extracellular coagulation of Limulus blood. *Bull. Johns Hopkins Hosp.* 115:265-274.

———. 1968. Clottable protein in Limulus: its localization and kinetics of its coagulation by endotoxin. *Thromb. Diath. Haemorrh.* 19:186-197.

Liebermeister, C. 1887. *Vorlesungen uber specielle pathologie und therapie*. Leipzig: Verlag von F.C.W. Vogel.

Lillywhite, H. B. 1970. Behavioral temperature regulation in the bullfrog, *Rana catesbeiana*. *Copeia* 158-168.

———. 1971. Thermal modulation of cutaneous mucus discharge as a determinant of evaporative water loss in the frog, *Rana catesbeiana*. *Z. vergl. Physiol.* 73:84-104.

Lipton, J. M. 1973. Thermosensitivity of medulla oblongata in control of body temperature. *Am. J. Physiol.* 224:890-897.

Lipton, J. M., and G. P. Trzcinka. 1976. Persistance of febrile response to pyrogens after PO/AH lesions in squirrel monkeys. *Am. J. Physiol.* 231:1638-1648.

Love, R., R. Z. Soriano, and R. J. Walsh. 1970. Effect of hyperthermia on normal and neoplastic cells in vitro. *Cancer Res.* 30:1525-1533.

Lowry, W. P. 1967. *Weather and Life: An Introduction to Biometeorology*. New York: Academic Press.

Luderitz, O., C. Galanos, V. Lehmann, M. Nurminen, E. T. Rietschel, G. Rosenfelder, M. Simon, and O. Westphal. 1973. Lipid A: Chemical structure and biological activity. *J. Infect. Dis.* 128(supp):S17-S29.

Lwoff, A. 1959. Factors influencing the evolution of viral diseases at the cellular level and in the organism. *Bact. Rev.* 23:109-124.

———. 1969. Death and transfiguration of a problem. *Bact. Rev.* 33:390-403.

Major, R. H. 1954. *A History of Medicine*, Vol. 1. Springfield: C. C. Thomas.

Malvin, M. D., L. K. Vaughn, and M. J. Kluger. 1978. Blood pressure in bacterially infected rabbits—effects of antipyretic drug therapy. *Fed. Proc.* 37:661.

Mandell, G. L. 1975. Effect of temperature on phagocytosis by human polymorphonuclear neutrophils. *Infect. Immun.* 12:221-223.

Marantz, S. A. 1969. *Physics*. New York: Benziger, Inc.

McCutchan, F. W., and C. L. Taylor. 1951. Respiratory heat exchange with varying temperature and humidity of inspired air. *J. Appl. Physiol.* 4:121-135.

Mears. G. J., K. E. Cooper, and W. L. Veale. 1977. The in vitro Limulus assay for detection and measurement of bacterial pyrogens. In *Drugs, Biogenic Amines and Body Temperature*, ed. K. E. Cooper, P. Lomax, and E. Schonbaum, pp. 122-128. Basel: S. Karger.

Meeuse, B.J.D. 1966. The voodoo lily. *Scient. Amer.* 215:80-87.

Mendelssohn, M. 1902. Recherches sur la thermotaxie des organismes unicellulaires. *J. de Physiol. et de Path. Gen.* 4:393-410.

Merriman, C. R., L. A. Pulliam, and R. F. Kampschmidt. 1977. Comparison of leukocytic pyrogen and leukocytic endogenous mediator. *Soc. Expt. Biol. Med., Proc.* 154:224-227.

Mills, S. H., and J. E. Heath. 1972a. Responses to thermal stimulation of the preoptic area in the house sparrow, *Passer domesticus*. *Am. J. Physiol.* 222:914-919.

Mills, S. H., and J. E. Heath. 1972b. Anterior hypothalamic/preoptic lesions impair normal thermoregulation in house sparrows. *Comp. Biochem. Physiol.* 43:125-129.

Milton, A. S., and M. J. Dascombe. 1977. Cyclic nucleotides in thermoregulation and fever. In *Drugs, Biogenic Amines and Body Temperature*, ed. K. E. Cooper, P. Lomax, and E. Schonbaum, pp. 129-135. Basel: S. Karger.

Milton, A. S., and S. Wendlandt. 1971. Effects on body temperature of prostaglandins of the A, E and F series on injection into the third ventricle of unanesthetized cats and rabbits. *J. Physiol.* (Lond.) 218:325-336.

Moore, D. M., S. F. Cheuk, J. D. Morton, R. D. Berlin, and W. B. Wood, Jr. 1970. Studies on the pathogenesis of fever. XVIII. Activation of leukocytes for pyrogen production. *J. Expt. Med.* 131:179-188.

Moore, D. M., P. S. Murphy, P. J. Chesney, and W. B. Wood, Jr. 1973. Studies of endogenous pyrogen by rabbit leukocytes. *J. Expt. Med.* 137:1263-1274.

Mudd, S., B. Locke, M. McCutcheon, and M. Strumia. 1929. On the mechanism of opsonin and bacteriotropin action. I. Correlation between changes in bacterial surface properties and in phagocytosis by sera of animals under immunization. *J. Expt. Med.* 49:779-795.

Muschenheim, C., D. R. Duerschrer, J. D. Hardy, and A. M. Stoll. 1943. Hypothermia in experimental infections. III. The effect of hypothermia on resistance to experimental pneumococcus infection. *J. Infect. Dis.* 72:187-196.

Myers, R. D., and J. E. Buckman. 1972. Deep hypothermia induced in the golden hamster by altering cerebral calcium levels. *Am. J. Physiol.* 223:1313-1318.

Myers, R. D., and M. Tytell. 1972. Fever: reciprocal shift in brain sodium to calcium ratio as the set-point temperature rises. *Science* 178:765-767.

Myers, R. D., and W. L. Veale. 1970. Body temperature: possible ionic mechanism in the hypothalamus controlling the set point. Science 170:95-97.

———. 1971. The role of sodium and calcium ions in the hypothalamus in the control of body temperature of the unanesthetized cat. *J. Physiol.* (Lond.) 212:411-430.

Myers, R. D., and T. L. Yaksh, 1971. Thermoregulation around a new 'set-point' established in the monkey by altering the ratio of sodium to calcium ions within the hypothalamus. *J. Physiol.* (Lond.) 218:609-633.

Myhre, K., M. Cabanac, and G. Myhre. 1977 Fever and behavioural temperature regulation in the frog *Rana esculenta*. *Acta Physiol. Scand.* 101:219-229.

Myhre, K., and H. T. Hammel. 1969. Behavioral regulation of internal-temperature in the lizard *Tiliqua scincoides*. *Am. J. Physiol.* 217:1490-1495.

Nadel, E. R., J. W. Mitchell, and J.A.J. Stolwijk. 1973. Differential thermal sensitivity in the human skin. *Pflugers Arch*. 340:71-76.

Nadel, E. R., J. W. Mitchell, B. Saltin, and J.A.J. Stolwijk. 1971. Peripheral modifications to the central drive for sweating. *J. Appl. Physiol*. 31:828-833.

Nagy, K. A., D. K. Odell, and R. S. Seymour. 1972. Temperature regulation by the inflorescence of philodendron. *Science* 178:1195-1197.

Nahas, G. G., M. L. Tannieres, and J. F. Lennon. 1971. Direct measurement of leukocyte motility: effects of pH and temperature. *Soc. Expt. Biol. Med., Proc.* 138:350-352.

Nauts, H. C., G. A. Fowler, and F. H. Bogatko. 1953. A review of the influence of bacterial infection and of bacterial products (Coley's toxins) on malignant tumors in man. *Acta Med. Scand.* (supp) 276:1-103.

Nielsen, B. 1974a. Actions of intravenous Ca^{++} and Na^{+} on body temperature in rabbits. *Acta Physiol. Scand.* 90:445-450.

———. 1974b. Effect of changes in plasma Na^{+} and Ca^{++} ion concentration on body temperature during exercise. *Acta Physiol. Scand.* 91:123-129.

Nielsen, B., G. Hansen, S. O. Jorgensen, and E. Nielsen. 1971. Thermoregulation in exercising man during dehydration and hyperhydration with water and saline. *Int. J. Biometeor.* 15:195-200.

Nielsen, B., P. Schwartz, and J. Alhede. 1973. Is fever in man reflected in changes in cerebrospinal-fluid concentrations of sodium and calcium ions? *Scan. J. Clin. and Lab. Invest.* 32:309-310.

Nistico, G., and E. Marley. 1973. Central effects of prostaglandin E_1 in adult fowls. *Neuropharmacol.* 12:1009-1016.

Nordlund, J. J., R. K. Root, and S. M. Wolff. 1970. Studies on the origin of human leukocyte pyrogen. *J. Expt. Med.* 131:727-743.

Nowotny, A. 1969. Molecular aspects of endotoxic reactions. *Bact. Rev.* 33:72-98.

Nutik, S. L. 1973. Posterior hypothalamic neurons responsive to preoptic region thermal stimulation. *J. Neurophysiol.* 36:238-249.

Overgaard, J. 1977. Effect of hyperthermia on malignant cells in vivo. *Cancer* 39:2637-2646.

Parratt, J. R., and R. M. Sturgess. 1974. The effect of indomethacin on the cardiovascular and metabolic responses to E. coli endotoxin in the cat. *Br. J. Pharmacol.* 50:177-183.

Payne, J. F. 1900. *Thomas Sydenham.* London: T. Fisher Unwin.

Pembrey, M. S. 1895. The effect of variations in external temperature upon the output of carbonic acid and the temperature of young animals. *J. Physiol.* (Lond.) 18:364-379.

Phelps, P., and D. Stanislaw. 1969. Polymorphonuclear leukocyte mobility in vitro. I. Effect of pH, temperature, ethyl alcohol and caffeine, using a modified Boyden chamber technique. *Arthritis and Rheumatism* 12:181-188.

Philipp-Dormston, W. K., and R. Seigert. 1974. Prostaglandins of the E and F series in rabbit cerebrospinal fluid during fever induced by Newcastle disease virus, *E. coli*-endotoxin, or endogenous pyrogen. *Med. Microbiol. Immunol.* 159:279-284.

———. 1975. Fever produced in rabbits by N^6O^2-dibutyrl adenosine 3′, 5′ cyclic monophosphate. *Experientia* 31. 471-472

Pirie, N. W. 1972. Degree of fact. *Science* 175:10.

Pittman, Q. J., W. L. Veale, A. W. Cockeram, and K. E. Cooper. 1976. Changes in body temperature produced by prostaglandins and pyrogens in the chicken. *Am. J. Physiol.* 230:1284-1287.

Pittman, Q. J., W. L. Veale, and K. E. Cooper. 1977. Effect of prostaglandin, pyrogen and noradrenaline, injected into the hypothalamus, on thermoregulation in newborn lambs. *Brain Res.* 128:473-483.

Ponder, E., and J. MacLeod. 1938. Oxygen consumption of white cells from peritoneal exudates. *Am. J. Physiol.* 123:420-423.

Porter, P. J., and E. H. Kass. 1962. Mediation by the central nervous system of the lethal action of bacterial endotoxin. *Clin. Res.* 10:185.

Ranson, S. W., and H. W. Magoun. 1939. The hypothalamus. *Ergebnisse Physiol.* 41:56-163.

Ratliff, F. 1967. Halden Keffer Hartline. *Science* 158:471-473.

Rautenberg, W., R. Necker, and B. May. 1972. Thermoregulatory responses of the pigeon to changes of the brain and the spinal cord temperatures. *Pflugers Arch.* 338:31-42.

Rawson, R. O., and K. P. Quick. 1972. Localization of intra-abdominal thermoreceptors in the ewe. *J. Physiol.* (Lond.) 222:665-677.

Reynolds, W. W. 1977. Fever and antipyresis in the bluegill sunfish, *Lepomis macrochirus*. *Comp. Biochem. Physiol.* 57C:165-167.

Reynolds, W. W., M. E. Casterlin, and J. B. Covert. 1976. Behavioural fever in teleost fishes. *Nature* 259:41-42.

———. 1978. Febrile responses of bluegill (*Lepomis macrochirus*) to bacterial pyrogens. *J. Thermal Biol.* 3:129-130.

Reynolds, W. W., and J. B. Covert. 1977. Behavioral fever in aquatic ectothermic vertebrates. In *Drugs, Biogenic Amines and Body Temperature*, ed. K. E. Cooper, P. Lomax, and E. Schonbaum, pp. 108-110. Basel: S. Karger.

Reynolds, W. W., J. B. Covert, and M. E. Casterlin. 1978. Febrile responses of goldfish *Carassius auratus* (L.) to *Aeromonas hydrophila* and to *Escherichia coli* endotoxin. *J. Fish Diseases* 1:271-273.

Reynolds, W. W., R. W. McCauley, M. E. Casterlin, and L. I. Crawshaw. 1976. Body temperatures of behaviorally thermoregulating largemouth blackbass (*Micropterus salmoides*). *Comp. Biochem. Physiol.* 54:461-463.

Richards, S. A. 1970. The biology and comparative physiology of thermal panting. *Biol. Rev.* 45:223-264.

Riedel, W., G. Siaplauras, and E. Simon. 1973. Intra-abdominal thermosensitivity in the rabbit as compared with spinal thermosensitivity. *Pflugers Arch.* 340:59-70.

Riedesel, M. L., J. L. Cloudsley-Thompson, and J. A. Cloudsley-Thompson. 1971. Evaporative thermoregulation in turtles. *Physiol. Zool.* 44:28-32.

Roberts, N. J., Jr., and R. T. Steigbigel. 1977. Hyperthermia and human leukocyte functions: effects on response of lymphocytes to mitogen and antigen and bactericidal capacity of monocytes and neutrophils. *Infect. and Immun.* 18:673-679.

Robertshaw, D., and C. N. Beier. 1977. The relationship between plasma levels of sodium and ionized calcium and thermoregulatory thresholds at different phases of the human menstrual cycle. *The Physiologist* 20(4):80.

Roitt, I. 1974. Essential Immunology. Oxford: Blackwell Scientific Publ.

Romer, A. S. 1966. *Vertebrate Paleontology*. Chicago: University of Chicago Press.

Root, R. K., and S. M. Wolff. 1968. Pathogenetic mechanisms in experimental immune fever. *J. Expt. Med.* 128:309-323.

Rosendorff, C., and J. J. Mooney. 1971. Central nervous system sites of action of a purified leucocyte pyrogen. *Am. J. Physiol.* 220:597-603.

Rowell, L. B. 1974. The cutaneous circulation. In *Physiology and Biophysics*, ed. T. C. Ruch and H. D. Patton, pp. 185-199. Philadelphia: W. B. Saunders Co.

Sadowski, B., and E. Szczepanska-Sadowska. 1974. The effect of calcium ions chelation and sodium ions excess in the cerebrospinal fluid on body temperature in conscious dogs. *Pflugers Arch.* 352:61-68.

Satinoff, E. 1972. Salicylate: action on normal body temperature in rats. *Science* 176:532-533.

Satinoff, E., G. N. McEwen, Jr., and B. A. Williams. 1976. Behavioral fever in newborn rabbits. *Science* 193:1139-1140.

Schmidt-Nielsen, K. 1972. How Animals Work. London: Cambridge University Press.

Schoener, E. P., and S. C. Wang. 1975. Observations on the central mechanism of acetylsalicylate antipyresis. *Life Sci.* 17:1063-1068.

Schreiner, H. J. 1936. Das Warmegefuhl nach calcium-injektionen. Inaug.-Diss., Gottingen.

Sebag, J., W. P. Reed, and R. C. Williams, Jr. 1977. Effect of temperature on bacterial killing by serum and by polymorphonuclear leukocytes. *Infect. Immun.* 16:947-954.

Seibert, F. B. 1923. Fever-producing substances found in some distilled waters. *Am. J. Physiol.* 67:90-104.

———. 1925. The cause of many febrile reactions following intravenous injections. I. *Am. J. Physiol.* 71:621-651.

Seoane, J. R., and A. C. Baile. 1973. Ionic changes in cerebrospinal fluid and feeding, drinking and temperature of sheep. *Physiol. Behav.* 10:915-923.

Sharp, F. R., and H. T. Hammel. 1972. Effects of fever on salivation response in the resting and exercising dog. *Am. J. Physiol.* 223:77-82.

Simon, E. 1974. Temperature regulation: the spinal cord as a site of extrahypothalamic thermoregulatory functions. *Rev. Physiol. Biochem. Pharmacol.* 71:1-76.

Smith, J. B., and A. L. Willis. 1971. Aspirin selectively inhibits prostaglandin production in human platelets. *Nature New Biology* 231:235-237.

Snapp, B. D., H. C. Heller, and S. M. Gospe, Jr., 1977. Hypothalamic thermosensitivity in California quail (*Lophortyx californicus*). *J. Comp. Physiol.* 117:345-357.

Snell, E. S. 1971. Endotoxin and the pathogenesis of fever. In *Microbial Toxins*, ed. S. Kadis, G. Weinbaum, and S. J. Ajl. Vol. V. *Bacterial Endotoxins*, pp. 277-340. New York: Academic Press.

Snell, E. S., and E. Atkins. 1968. The mechanisms of fever. In *The Biological Basis of Medicine*, ed. E. E. Bittar and N. Bittar, pp. 397-419. New York: Academic Press.

Sobocinska, J., and J. E. Greenleaf. 1976. Cerebrospinal fluid [Ca^{2+}] and rectal temperature response during exercise in dogs. *Am. J. Physiol.* 230:1416-1419.

Solomon, H. A., A. Berk, M. Theiler, and C. L. Clay. 1926. Use of sodoku in the treatment of general paralysis. A preliminary report. *Arch. Intern. Med.* 38:391-404.

Speirer, C. 1931. Die unspezifische behandlung der gonorrhoe mit pyrifer. *Derm. Wschr.* 92:13-17.

Splawinski, J. A., E. Zacny, and Z. Gorka. 1977. Fever in rats after intravenous *E. coli* endotoxin administration. *Pflugers Arch.* 368:125-128.

Stedman's Medical Dictionary. 1972. Baltimore: The Williams and Wilkins Co.

Stitt, J. T. 1973. Prostaglandin E_1 fever induced in rabbits. *J. Physiol.* (Lond.) 232:163-179.

Stitt, J. T., and J. D. Hardy. 1975. Microelectrophoresis of PGE_1 onto single units in the rabbit hypothalamus. *Am. J. Physiol.* 229:240-245.

Stricker, E. M., and F. R. Hainsworth. 1970. Evaporative cooling in the rat: effects of dehydration. *Can. J. Physiol. and Pharmacol.* 48:18-27.

Strouse, S. 1909. Experimental studies on pneumococcus infections. *J. Expt. Med.* 11:743-761.

Suit, H. D., and M. Shwayder. 1974. Hyperthermia: potential as an anti-tumor agent. *Cancer* 34:122-129.

Suzuki, K. 1967. Application of heat to cancer chemotherapy —experimental studies. *Nagoya J. Med. Sci.* 30:1-21.

Tabatabai, M. 1972. Respiratory and cardiovascular responses resulting from cooling the medulla oblongata in cats. *Am. J. Physiol.* 223:8-12.

Taylor, F. S. 1942. The origin of the thermometer. *Annals of Science* 5:129-156.

Teisner, B., and S. Haahr. 1974. Poikilothermia and susceptibility of suckling mice to Coxsackie B1 virus. *Nature* 247:568.

Templeton, J. R. 1970. Reptiles. In *Comparative Physiology of Ther-*

moregulation, ed. G. C. Whittow, pp. 167-221. New York: Academic Press.

Thompson, D. W. 1942. *On Growth and Form*. New York: Macmillan Co.

Thompson, G. E., and J.A.F. Stevenson. 1965. The temperature responses of the male rat to treadmill exercise, and the effect of anterior hypothalamic lesions. *Can. J. Physiol. Pharm.* 43:279-287.

Toms, G. L., J. A. Davies, C. G. Woodward, C. Sweet, and H. Smith. 1977. The relation of pyrexia and nasal inflammatory response to virus levels in nasal washings of ferrets infected with influenza viruses of differing virulence. *Br. J. Exp. Path.* 58:444-458.

Turlejska-Stelmasiak, E. 1974. The influence of dehydration on heat dissipation mechanisms in the rabbit. *J. Physiol.* (Paris) 68:5-15.

United States Pharmacopeia. 1975. Easton, Pa.: Mack.

Vander, A. J., J. H. Sherman, and D. S. Luciano. 1975. *Human Physiology, The Mechanisms of Body Function.* New York: McGraw-Hill.

Vane, J. R. 1971. Inhibition of prostaglandin synthesis as a mechanism of action for aspirin-like drugs. *Nature New Biology* 231:232-235.

van Miert. A.S.J.P.A.M., J. A. van Essen, and G. A. Tromp. 1972. The antipyretic effect of pyrazolone derivatives and salicylates on fever induced with leukocytic or bacterial pyrogen. *Archs. Int. Pharmacodyn. Ther.* 197:388-391.

van Miert, A.S.J.P.A.M., and J. Frens. 1968. The reaction of different animal species to bacterial pyrogens. *Zbl. Vet. Med.* 15:532-543.

Vaughn, L. K., H. A. Bernheim, and M. J. Kluger. 1974. Fever in the lizard *Dipsosaurus dorsalis*. *Nature* 252:473-474.

Vaughn, L. K., and M. J. Kluger. 1977. Fever and survival in bacterially infected rabbits. *Fed. Proc.* 36(3):511.

Veale, W. L., and K. E. Cooper. 1975. Comparison of sites of action of prostaglandin E and leucocyte pyrogen in brain. In *Temperature Regulation and Drug Action,* ed. P. Lomax, pp. 218-226. Basel: S. Karger.

Wagner, R. R. 1953. Production of fever by influenza viruses. IV. Tolerance to mumps and influenza pyrogens. *Soc. Exp. Biol. Med., Proc.* 83:612-615.

Wagner, R. R., I. L. Bennett, Jr., and V. S. LeQuire. 1949. The production of fever by influenza viruses. I. Factors influencing the febrile response to single injections of virus. *J. Expt. Med.* 90:321-334.

Wagner-Jauregg, J. 1927. The treatment of dementia paralytica by malaria inoculation. In *Nobel Lectures: Physiology or Medicine, 1922-1941,* pp. 159-169. New York: Elsevier Publ. Co.

Watson, S. W., R. W. Guenther, and R. R. Rucker. 1954. A virus disease of sockeye salmon: interim report *U.S. Fish Wildl. Serv. Sci. Rep. Fish.* 138:36 pp.

Webster, A.J.F. 1974. Adaptation to the cold. In *Environmental Physiology*, Vol. 7, ed. D. Robertshaw, pp. 71-106. Baltimore: University Park Press.

Weinberg, E. D. 1974. Iron and susceptibility to infectious disease. *Science* 184:952-956.

———. 1978. Iron and infection. *Microbiol. Rev.* 42:45-66.

Wekstein, D. R., and J. F. Zolman. 1968. Sympathetic control of homeothermy in the young chick. *Am. J. Physiol.* 214:908-912.

Wernstedt, W. 1927. Introduction to Wagner-Jauregg's Nobel Lecture. In *Nobel Lectures: Physiology or Medicine, 1922-1941*, pp. 155-158. New York: Elsevier Publ. Co.

White, F. N. 1976. The role of the cardiovascular system in thermoregulation. In *The Biology of the Reptilia*, ed. C. Gans and W. R. Dawson, pp. 312-317. New York: Academic Press.

Willies, G. H., C. J. Woolf, and C. Rosendorff. 1976. The effect of an inhibitor of adenylate cyclase on the development of pyrogen, prostaglandin and cyclic AMP fevers in the rabbit. *Pflugers Arch.* 376:177-181.

Winter, C. A. and G. W. Nuss. 1963. Pyretogenic effects of bacterial lipopolysaccaharide and the assay of antipyretic drugs in the rat. *Tox. App. Pharmac.* 5:247-256.

Wit, A., and S. C. Wang. 1968. Temperature-sensitive neurons in preoptic/anterior hypothalamic region: actions of pyrogens and acetylsalicylate. *Am. J. Physiol.* 215:1160-1169.

Wolff, S. M., J. H. Mulholland, S. B. Ward, M. Rubenstein, and P. D. Mott. 1965. Effect of 6-mercaptopurine on endotoxin tolerance. *J. Clin. Invest.* 44:1402-1409.

Woodbury, D. M., and E. Fingl. 1975. Analgesic-antipyretics, anti-inflammatory agents, and drugs employed in the therapy of gout. In *The Pharmacological Basis of Therapeutics,* ed. L. S. Goodman and A. Gilman, pp. 325-358. New York: Macmillan Co.

Woolf, C. J., G. H. Willies, H. Laburn, and C. Rosendorff. 1975.

Pyrogen and prostaglandin fever in the rabbit. I. Effects of salicylate and the role of cyclic AMP. *Neuropharmacol.* 14:397-403.

Wunderlich, C. A. 1871. *On the Temperature in Diseases: A Manual of Medical Thermometry.* London: The New Sydenham Society.

Wunnenberg, W., and J. D. Hardy. 1972. Response of single units of the posterior hypothalamus to thermal stimulation. *J. Appl. Physiol.* 33:547-552.

Yokai, Y. 1969. Effect of heat and cold stress on thermal responses to antipyretic drugs. *Fed. Proc.* 28:1115-1117.

Yost, R. M., Jr. 1950. Sydenham's philosophy of science. *Osiris.* 9:84-104.

Young, N. S., L. Levin, and R. A. Prendergast. 1972. An invertebrate coagulation system activated by endotoxin: evidence for enzymatic mediation. *J. Clin. Invest.* 51:1790-1797.

Index

LIBRARY OF CONGRESS CATALOGING IN PUBLICATION DATA

Kluger, Matthew J 1946-
Fever, its biology, evolution, and function.

Includes index.
1. Fever. 2. Body temperature—Regulation.
3. Infection. 4. Physiology, Comparative.
I. Title.
RB129.K57 616′.047 79-83998
ISBN 0-691-08234-0